MW00587081

Safe in a Midwife's Hands

Birthing Traditions from Africa to the American South

Linda Janet Holmes

MAD CREEK BOOKS, AN IMPRINT OF
THE OHIO STATE UNIVERSITY PRESS
COLUMBUS

Copyright © 2023 by Linda Janet Holmes.
All rights reserved.
Published by Mad Creek Books, an imprint of The Ohio State University Press.

Library of Congress Cataloging-in-Publication Data available online at https://catalog.loc.gov
LCCN: 2022051159

Identifiers: ISBN 978-0-8142-5866-8 (paper); ISBN 978-0-8142-8279-3 (ebook)

Cover design by Nathan Putens
Text design by Juliet Williams
Type set in Adobe Minion Pro

∞ The paper used in this publication meets the minimum requirements of the American National Standard for Information Sciences—Permanence of Paper for Printed Library Materials. ANSI Z39.48-1992.

Advance Praise for *Safe in a Midwife's Hands*

"Building on forty years of skillfully listening to Black midwives, Holmes guides us on a stirring journey across continents, customs, and generations to illuminate the rich diasporic traditions of midwifery."

—Wangui Muigai, Brandeis University

"This is essential reading for all who respect and honor the tradition of midwifery. Catching babies is a physical, emotional, and spiritual art."

—Byllye Avery, founder, Black Women's Health Imperative

"For countless generations, midwives have been a steady support to women, a stabilizing force for the family, and trusted leaders in their communities. Hope resides in their hands and within the pages of Linda Janet Holmes's fascinating exploration of the birthing traditions of Black women from Alabama to their roots on the African continent. *Safe in a Midwife's Hands* is a must-read on issues at the intersection of racial and reproductive justice and a celebration of the enduring wisdom of Black women."

—Dr. Natalia Kanem, executive director, United Nations Population Fund

"*Safe in a Midwife's Hands* is a passionate, beautifully written account of the under-researched history of Black midwives on the African continent and in the American South. It makes an important contribution to our understanding of African retentions among African Americans and of the life-sustaining birthing justice movement here and around the globe. This heartfelt book makes visible Linda Holmes's decades-long commitment to telling our stories of healing and resistance."

—Beverly Guy-Sheftall, founding director of the Women's Research and Resource Center and Anna Julia Cooper Professor of Women's Studies, Spelman College

Safe in a Midwife's Hands

CONTENTS

ILLUSTRATIONS

PROLOGUE

Midwives taught me how to listen just like they listened to know when "time come for folk to get born." Midwives also taught me how to talk to God. All kinds of trouble can rise up when bringing life into the world in a one-room unlit cabin with no heat, as Alabama midwives told me. That's when midwives said they be talking to God, just like they be talking to any other man.

In 1981, when my work interviewing midwives began in Alabama, I spent more time with Rosie Aaron Smith on the porch of her home than I did with any of the other 50 midwives whose stories I recorded in Alabama.

Whenever I needed to sit with Miss Rosie, I knew the 85-year-old retired midwife would be sitting outdoors like midwives used to do when waiting for someone to take them out to care for the mother or "wait on the mother," as Miss Rosie would say. I never called to let Miss Rosie know I was coming, but she was always there.

Because Rosie lived alone in her three-room house built just across from her daughter's trailer, which seemed to be permanently parked in the yard, I could go straight to talking to Miss Rosie without having to greet or chat with others.

When Rosie spoke, her words floated into the Alabama heat and released a soft breeze that felt like a seductive goddess in the woods cooling the air. On Rosie's porch, which connected a front porch, back porch, and side porch, she would look out over toward her garden and say things like, "Don't need no fertilizer to grow this corn, just hum."

I learned from Rosie that hums also carried the pain and sorrow that marked enslavement, Jim Crow, and struggle like in the '60s when Black men and women sat on their front porches with guns to protect their families. And through all those times, midwives like Rosie Smith helped Black babies to get born.

While sitting on her front porch saying goodbye, Miss Rosie let me know that I would see her again and that the work I was doing would continue. On my last visit with Miss Rosie after interviewing midwives in 1981, Miss Rosie was wearing the everyday cotton polka-dotted brown dress adorned with buttons that I always saw her wearing. Her clothes, her porch, the house that she helped her sons to build looked worn, but the strength of her spirit guided me in the writing of this book. This book celebrates Rosie Aaron Smith and all the midwives who've been kind enough to share their stories with me.

MY JOURNEY

When I gave birth at St. Joseph's Hospital in Paterson, New Jersey, in 1976, I had no idea that my childbirth experience would launch a lifetime of work. Forty-five years later, I remain committed to activism and write in support of a growing birthing justice movement that aims to end inequities in birthing care and outcomes. I dedicate the stories in this book to that movement.

The fire I bring to this work still burns from my engagement in the 1960s Black student revolutionary movement. On the Rutgers University campus, I was among the Black students who raised our fists in making demands that challenged structural racism, the abysmal lack of Black faculty and classes focusing on Black history, and Black students' underrepresentation in the student population at this state-funded institution. Preparing for giving birth six years later felt like readying myself for a Black Power march on campus, but this time, the demands centered on seizing the power to make choices about my childbirth experience.

To prepare for childbirth, my partner Welton Smith and I took classes with Elisabeth Bing, known as the "mother of Lamaze," in her apartment on Manhattan's Upper East Side. Smith, a journalist and poet, was widely recognized for capturing the spirit of Malcolm X in his poem first published in *Black Fire,* edited by the revolutionary poet Amiri Baraka. As we prepared to give birth to our daughter, Ajoa Ghana Frisco Tashi Smith, we were the only Black couple in the Lamaze classes, where we learned breathing techniques for relaxation, ways to negotiate having husbands in the delivery room, and how to avoid unnecessary drugs and technological interventions.

Despite my preparation and determination to have my wishes respected, doctors administered Pitocin, a drug used to stimulate labor, and ordered an epidural, a procedure that injects a local anesthesia into the mother. In an act of self-empowerment, I refused to agree to an epidural unless my partner could be in the delivery room to provide emotional support. We also convinced the labor and delivery room nurses to agree to keep champagne chilled in the staff refrigerator for a celebration of Ghana's birth. That's when a nurse told me that I was the first in the hospital to request rooming with a newborn so that I could breastfeed with ease on demand. After this birth experience where I felt disempowered, I emerged as an activist who became part of a growing movement that focused on increasing access to birthing care that respected women's choices.

What I didn't know then, but later learned, is that many of "the best practices" that Lamaze classes promote are traditions that midwives support. Remaining active during labor, being awake and aware for birthing, using alternative upright birthing positions, and creating a welcoming environment that encourages women and others to gather to provide comfort throughout the birthing process are the hallmarks of traditional midwife practices from time immemorial. The African continent, the cradle of humanity, provides the earliest examples of how midwives were the caretakers of rituals celebrating the birth event.

This book begins with the stories of traditional midwives in Kenya, Ghana, and Ethiopia who describe timeless birthing traditions grounded in African religion and culture. While governmental agencies differentiate midwives who acquire their skills through apprenticeships from those who obtain their skills through formal educational programs in academic settings, a growing number of midwife organizations around the world increasingly focus on the commonalities that midwives share in their ways of caring during the birth event.

What became a lifetime of supporting midwifery practices began with full-time work at the University of Medicine and Dentistry in Newark, New Jersey (UMDNJ). While still a breastfeeding mom, I joined the UMDNJ nurse midwife faculty and provided administrative support, which created a rare opportunity to listen to midwife stories at weekly staff meetings as they described their work caring mostly for inner-city Black women at a teaching hospital's maternity care clinic. In the late '70s, I taught the first class offered within the midwife educational program that focused on increasing awareness of medical racism and provided examples of injustices Black women face when seeking health care within medical institutions. Of course, I told my personal birthing story.

When working with the nurse midwife program as an educational administrative assistant, I frequently accompanied Teresa Marsico, the program director, when she met with the chairperson of the Department of Obstetrics and Gynecology at the medical school. I seldom spoke and usually scribbled notes while remembering that the state of New Jersey had built the medical school on grounds that required decimating Black neighborhoods (now recognized as one of the underlying causes of the 1967 Newark Rebellion). At the time, a Black infant in Newark was more likely to die during birth than in any other major city in the country.

A decade after construction began on University Hospital, which became part of the academic medical center and replaced the city of Newark's Martland Hospital, I learned firsthand that deeply seated biases were still harbored by those in high-ranking positions at the newly established UMDNJ.

Marsico and I dreaded the closed-door meetings in his office because the chair of the Department, Dr. K., delighted in interjecting abusive sexist remarks into the conversation. "If you want to get a woman to go into labor, just stick a hot iron rod up her vagina," he often said, like a guy enjoying telling a dirty joke at the bar. I later learned that at one point, the American College of Obstetrics and Gynecology named him their spokesperson for public relations. Dr. K. also believed that most women who could afford to seek care from a doctor would seldom choose a midwife as her caregiver.

In an earlier encounter with him, while I was a master's student studying public administration at Rutgers University, Dr. K. tore up a survey instrument I had designed to collect input from these women, who often were treated as no more than "teaching material" for medical students. Growing up, I heard community members refer to Newark's Martland Hospital, where many of Newark's indigent women gave birth, as a "horse-pital." About the women now giving birth at what later became the medical center at UMDNJ, Dr. K. looked me straight in the eyes and said that because they were unmarried and most of them were alcoholics or on drugs, they wouldn't know anything about family-centered maternity care, and they wouldn't be interested in completing my survey.

I recently supported protests led by feminists and other activists in New York that resulted in the removal of the Central Park monument to Dr. James Marion Sims, known as the "father of gynecology." Sims ruthlessly experimented on enslaved Black women without anesthesia in Montgomery, Alabama, but some medical schools and medical associations continue to tout his exploitations as a success story. A Sims statue still stands on the Capitol lawn in Montgomery, even as numerous Confederate monuments tumbled in response to the Black Lives Matter movement.

While the monument to Sims still stands, public health officials decimated the practices of hundreds of thousands of traditional Black midwives across the South in the 1970s. Public health officials ended midwife practices when court rulings and federal legislation forced states to increase access to hospital-based medical care and the civil rights struggle ended Jim Crow segregation. In 2021 there are no monuments in Alabama honoring the hundreds of thousands of Black midwives who contributed to caring for and saving the lives of countless women, Black and white. A collective of Black women artists are erecting a monument to Lucy, Anarcha, and Betsey, who Sims ruthlessly experimented on in 1845.

In 1981, with support from an independent fellowship from the National Endowment for the Humanities, I moved with my four-year-old daughter and her dad to Alabama, where we lived for six months in order to interview a last generation of traditional Black midwives. The medical professions labeled Black midwives as necessary evils, because decades after Jim Crow segregation became illegal, inequities in birthing outcomes continue (then and still now) to be rooted in unequal treatment that Black women have received from doctors, as studies continue to document.

In Alabama, I collected stories from midwives whose friendships continued for years after I left Alabama. When I returned to New Jersey, I decided to leave the nurse midwife program at the University of Medicine and Dentistry of New Jersey, UMDNJ, when the American College of Nurse Midwives refused to integrate the history and contributions of Black, Indigenous, or immigrant midwives into the educational curriculum for midwifery students. At the time, the chairperson of the American College of Nurse Midwives Archives Committee also refused to accept the tapes of interviews I'd recorded with Alabama's Black lay midwives as a gift because she said that the mission of the college focused on nurse midwives only. Those interviews are now part of the emerging Smith College collection on Black women activists, midwives, and health care workers and are the backbone of this book.

Forty years after interviewing midwives in Alabama, I traveled independently to Kenya, Ethiopia, and Ghana, where once again I sat down with traditional midwives to record their stories. I selected countries where there were midwives who sustained timeless birthing traditions or who were familiar with these practices because their ancestors had passed them on to them. I also chose these places because nurse midwives whom I met at the UMDNJ worked with traditional midwives. The contacts they generously provided helped me arrange interviews with some of the midwives in this book. The questions I asked midwives on the Continent are rooted in the Alabama midwife stories. I also asked the questions that I thought the Alabama midwives might have asked if they could.

On the Continent, midwives talked about traditions that were grounded in African religions, which included chants and invocations. Black midwives in Alabama had shared Christian prayer, hums, and scripture, which resonated with the practices of some of the traditional midwives on the Continent.

On the Continent, "being born in the house" meant being wrapped in the strength of ancestral traditions. In Kenya, midwives looked to the sky to determine an infant's name, using the amount of light or the sun or moon's position to make the determination. Many midwives also described the birthing hut as a welcoming space, unlike a facility or hospital where mothers are routinely separated from loved ones and women may be unable to adhere to their religiously based birthing traditions. In Alabama, a midwife told me that she sold her cow to have enough money to give birth in the hospital. "I had as much pain in the hospital as I had at home," she said. "I decided not to go to the hospital for the next one."

In Hampton, Virginia, where I now live, I learned from Nichole Wardlaw, a Black nurse midwife who heads Jamii Birth and Wellness Services, that she was the only Black nurse midwife supporting women who wanted a home birth in the area in 2022. At the time, one other Black nurse midwife worked at the naval hospital in nearby Portsmouth. Wardlaw confirmed that now a growing number of women in Virginia are choosing to give birth at home with a midwife, but they often face challenges finding a midwife.

In the Virginia chapter, I include the stories of currently practicing Black midwives and other birth workers to demonstrate how some of the traditions described by Black midwives in Alabama and on the Continent continue. For example, Virginia midwives discuss how they focus on the overall well-being of the woman and her family in culturally specific ways. Midwives also explain how their wholistic practices address growing concerns about medical inequities and injustices.

In Virginia, the descendants of midwives and women who came into the world through the hands of midwives offer their midwifery tributes, while others describe the challenges they faced when giving birth in the hospital. Alongside these stories, I offer my own reflections on a lifetime of experiences in the birthing justice movement. This book also invites readers to extrapolate from and integrate into their own birthing experiences some of the timeless birthing traditions described by midwives here. Throughout the book, the influence of place, ancestry, gender, politics, racism, and sexism provide context for the birthing stories that are found in this collage.

As I prepared to leave Ghana in 2019, I thought back on the coldness and the inappropriate interventions that I believe shaped my birthing story 45 years ago. A few days before my returning flight to Virginia, I met with doctors and researchers at the Mampong Centre for Plant Medicine Research in Mampong-Akwapim, Ghana, which has studied and produced plant medicines since 1976. Researchers described that even when the benefits of herbal medicines are scientifically studied and found useful, women face challenges when seeking to access plant-based medicines as part of their prenatal care.

When meeting with Baffour Osei Akoto at the Centre, I told him of the United States' growing birthing justice movement. Working to address long-standing health disparities, I explained how doulas, midwives, and women are in the forefront of that movement. Even so, I worried that traditions sustained by traditional midwives—traditions that promoted interconnecting physical, mental, and spiritual well-being— might not survive as a key element of this birthing justice movement.

Akoto smiled and immediately answered my question with a question. "Didn't you just tell me that aspects of the African traditions of midwifery survived the Middle Passage, enslavement, and Jim Crow?" I laughed and embraced a newfound optimism.

Midwives, doulas, mothers, midwife descendants, and activists answer that question in "Hampton to Charlottesville: Rebirthing Midwife Traditions," the last chapter of this book. Along with asking them these questions, I talked with them about how I refused to comply with the rules and regulations promoted by doctors and nurses when I gave birth. And I told them that I applauded the traditional midwives of African descent in Alabama who rejected the rules that threatened them in order to sustain the traditions passed on to them by their ancestors (some of whom were born on the Continent).

In Africa and in many Indigenous cultures, women viewed birthing as a time of spiritual ascendance. These and other birthing practices survived in villages where I discussed traditions with today's birth workers. Now the midwives I talked to on the Continent described how the use of massage, plant-based medicines, and an array of religiously based traditions are being degraded and no longer allowed by some of the Western-trained doctors and nurses who supervise their practice. I realized that these regulations threatened the core of traditional midwife practices on the Continent just as they once had in the American South, where traditional midwife practices once were ubiquitous. I promised the midwives I met that I was not there to simply record stories for a university library collection. I was there to champion their voices so they could be more widely heard and appreciated for their contributions, and so that together we could champion the preservation of these birthing traditions.

Looking back, I can see now that my birthing experience more than four decades ago in a busy Paterson, New Jersey, hospital with a doctor I barely knew was the beginning of a lifelong involvement in the birthing justice movement. Little did I know at the time, though, that my experience would drive me not just to learn more about the origins of alternative birthing methods and traditions in the States, but that it would one day take me on a transatlantic journey to learn firsthand about birthing cultures from time immemorial.

NOTE ON THE TEXT

Rather than place the chapters in this book on a linear time-line, I organized them to emphasize how midwife stories from Africa, Alabama, and Virginia are interconnected in an unbroken circle of birthing traditions and practices.

Throughout this book, I use the terms *traditional midwife* and *midwife* interchangeably. I define a traditional midwife (or midwife) as a woman who supports mothers before, during, and after childbirth and integrates culturally based traditions and spiritual practices into the birthing experience. A traditional midwife is often an herbalist or healer who is respected in her community as a holistic caregiver and advisor. The World Health Organization defines a woman who has acquired her skills in providing birthing care through apprenticeships and experience as a Traditional Birth Attendant (TBA). Unfortunately, TBAs are often viewed as being in the lower ranks of medical hierarchies even when their birthing outcomes are equal to or better than those of accredited and professionally trained health care providers.

The midwives I interviewed for this book include women who apprenticed with experienced elders assisting women in their villages and communities at birth, as well as women who were introduced to culturally based birthing traditions through their own birth experiences or through the birth experiences of women they knew.

When meeting midwives in Africa, I frequently introduced myself by my first name and seldom referred to my academic studies in public health or anthropology. I told every midwife I met, however, "I am a mother, grandmother, and writer who's worked to support midwife practices for decades."

When I told midwives that I traveled alone from the US to meet them and record their stories, their gratitude was palpable and required no translation. Water filled their eyes as I told them that some of the practices that they described had been safely preserved by Black midwives in the US for centuries.

I identify the majority of the midwives I interviewed by their real names. In Kenya, I changed the names of the midwives that I interviewed as requested by the agency who made it possible for me to meet them and record their stories. The two Kenya chapters are the only chapters where midwives are identified by pseudonymous first names only. In the remaining chapters, all of the midwives and others are identified by their real first and last names.

During interviews, sometimes male and female family members volunteered to serve as interpreters. I have preserved the stories of the midwives in their own words, but I have edited some interview transcripts for clarity and repetition.

Personal savings and a last-minute GoFundMe drive supported my work in Kenya, Ethiopia, and Ghana. A fellowship from the National Endowment for the Humanities funded my travel and living expenses in Alabama. While I was living in Hampton, a Virginia Humanities Fellowship funded my work to continue documenting midwife stories.

I began thinking about writing this book more than 40 years ago, wondering how far back I would be able to trace this lineage of midwifery practices. Decades later, I've learned that midwives of African descent in the US have sustained many of the timeless birthing traditions and practices their people first cultivated in Africa, the cradle of humanity where midwife practices were first born.

CHAPTER 1

Korogocho

Massage Techniques, Spiritual Cleansings, Urban Gardens

Four hundred years after the landing of the *White Lion,* a ship carrying the first Africans to their enslavement in English-occupied colonial America, the nation paused for collective remembrance of the horrors, acts of resistance, and resilience that marked the experience of African Americans then and now. But no one mentioned African American midwives in any of the celebrations that I attended at Fort Monroe, previously known as Point Comfort, on the Chesapeake Bay in Hampton, Virginia, just a few miles from my home.

My work in Africa began five months before marking the historic arrival of enslaved Africans that made possible the building of what became the United States. My flight landed in Nairobi, Kenya, just months before Nana Akufo-Addo, Ghana's then president, declared 2019 the "Year of Return" for those of African descent scattered across the diaspora. On the flight, a young environmental activist spoke to me about his work with a growing international movement that included young Africans across the Continent clamoring for initiatives to address the increasing impact of climate change that challenged our "linear models based on take, make and dispose."

In the minutes that it took the plane to land, our conversation escalated into what reminded me of a heated community organizer meeting among comrades building coalitions. Michael was there to attend the Fourth Session of the United Nations Environment Assembly on "Innovative Solutions for Environment Challenges" scheduled to begin the next day. My own work to document the practices of traditional midwives would follow one day of rest after the international flight. In Nairobi, I would be meeting with traditional midwives to learn how they employed massage and therapeutic touch in their practice.

Interviews began in Kenya because a friend urging me to reach out to the African Population and Health Research Center in Kenya for assistance with interpretation and translation services led to me beginning my interviews for this book in Nairobi. Having imagined beginning interviews in a village in the mountains of rural Kenya, the Foundation staff surprised me by suggesting that I begin my interviews with midwives in one of Nairobi's oldest and largest informal settlements, Korogocho, which is the Swahili word for "shoulder to shoulder."

In the 1960s, following the revolutionary overthrow of a British colonial rule that re-enforced white privilege, an estimated 200,000 migrants including Kikuyu, Luo, and Luhya peoples and various ethnic and religious groups abandoned environmentally friendly mud-walled and grass-thatched-roof huts seeking new opportunities in Nairobi. Unable to find housing, migrants huddled together in the place now called Korogocho. Determined, new urbanites recycled discarded tin, scrap metal, iron sheets, and cardboard to create Korogocho on the 1.5 kilometers of land they claimed next to Nairobi's largest dumpsite; although their numbers have dwindled, some midwives continue to be caregivers in Korogocho. While others spotlight the poverty and difficult living conditions found in these communities, I looked forward to stepping into a settlement that I imagined might remind me of stereotypic descriptions of Newark, New Jersey. What others might have called a slum, I embraced as my beloved church community.

As the van driver weaved in and out of traffic, I worried: Would the Korogocho midwives I was scheduled to meet be familiar with the traditional birthing practices of midwives who had provided care in villages generations ago? In 2013 the Kenyan government made hospital-based maternity care free, and government campaigns encourage all women to deliver their babies in hospital; given their proximity in Korogocho to a hospital, I wondered how midwives even fit into this picture. And I worried whether midwives would be willing to share any of their traditional practices with me even if they could. As an outsider who didn't speak their language, would I be trusted? Would they reveal to a stranger the ways of their grandmothers who previously served their villages as midwives?

In 1981, when I moved from New Jersey to Alabama to interview African American midwives about the traditions they sustained in their practices before the state prohibited the issuance of lay-midwife permits, I worried about being an outsider. In Alabama, I quickly realized that not only did the midwives welcome an opportunity to tell their stories, they welcomed the opportunity to tell their stories to *me*. Several midwives told me how glad they were that I was Black. "Usually, the women doing this kind of work are white," one midwife explained. Now I wondered what expectations the African midwives I was scheduled to meet that morning would have about me.

In Korogocho, from the moment I stepped off the van, I felt welcomed. Women and children rushed out to meet me and the translator to accompany us on our walk to the house of the first midwife on my schedule. The hip-hop music blasting from speakers and graffiti on the walls reminded me of a block party in my community at home. Taking my time to keep my balance as I stepped over the cardboard covering the open gutters and sewers, I knew to avoid looking down as I walked. Having learned to walk similar narrow pathways with grace when visiting healers in Ibadan, Nigeria, I focused on what was ahead, like the beauty in the abstract graffiti art that popped up on storefronts and the colorful African cloth hanging in doorways. And then I saw a woman walking toward me; I immediately knew she was the midwife even before she spoke (see figure 1.1).

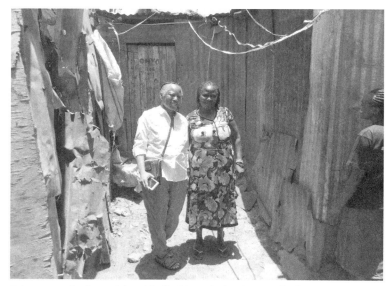

FIGURE 1.1. Author with midwife Naomi, the first midwife interviewed in Korogocho

"I am so glad you have come all the way from the United States to talk to me," the midwife, Naomi, said, welcoming me in a tone that I felt would comfort a mother in labor. Wearing a Sunday church outfit with color-coordinated blue flip-flops accenting the patches of blue sky in her dress, her style and splendor defied the Korogocho statistics that highlighted poverty, crime, high HIV rates, assaults, and sexual abuse including rape.

Seeing mothers with babies gathered at her door, now just steps away, there was no sign needed to know that this was Naomi's place. The dirt floor that I stepped onto in entering her home showed marks of being so recently swept that I immediately wanted to remove my rusty, worn red sandals before entering. But that would've made me look like an American tourist or a leftover 1960s hippie, so instead I quickly closed my eyes and went into a meditative space where I could focus on and feel the sanctity within the place.

As Naomi squatted to sit on a small wooden stool—one that a midwife would use when catching a baby—she pointed to the room's largest chair, covered with boldly colored upholstery and missing one armrest; I immediately knew that it was reserved for special guests, and I was honored to take that seat. As the interview began, children and chickens freely walked in and out of our conversation. During the interview, I listened to Naomi like a newcomer at a village gathering for a storytelling by a respected wise person or elder. As I watched women coming and going and others lingering at her door throughout our conversation, Naomi explained that some of the women were there to buy herbs, and others were pregnant women there for a massage. Naomi lightly touched my abdomen to demonstrate her massage technique.

Born in Migori, more than 200 miles from Nairobi, Naomi still makes regular visits home, which requires a six-hour bus trip to reach her village. Naomi began by describing how her knowledge of herbal medicines and massage techniques came both from the formal training she had received and her apprenticeship with her mother, a renowned midwife in Naomi's childhood village.

Naomi explained that when providing a pregnant woman a massage, she often also recommended taking a protective bath with herbal leaves. As a holistic caregiver and urban gardener, Naomi said she took advantage of those moments while relaxing mothers with her hands to explain to them the importance of eating an abundance of African vegetables as well as drinking teas made from plants which would help them build up their strength (Naomi made these teas from the plants that grow wildly at the edge of the settlement). I was reminded of how my beautician would often discuss a range of beauty products with me while doing my hair.

NAOMI: *So here, we have a variety of different types of vegetables. So we have amaranth, we have spider web leaves, we have pumpkin leaves, cabbage leaves, and we have the pigeon pea leaves that are normally eaten. Then we also have other wild leaves that people find in the community to eat. So, there are all kinds of varieties of traditional vegetables.*

While many of the midwives I met on the Continent explained how their mothers and elders in the community had introduced them to timeless traditions surrounding birth along with sharing their wisdom about the benefits of massage and plant medicine, Naomi had integrated lessons learned from apprenticing with her mother with the knowledge she obtained in a formal training program for traditional birth attendants.

NAOMI: *The whites came in a project at Gwedhi Masai. The year was '82. So we used to go like someone going to college for seven months. You are taught the using of herbal medicine. If you do this, it will do that. If a mother does not go into labor quickly, there is medicine to give her and the baby comes out safe. So, I stayed there for seven months while attending the college. I learned many things from training—medicines and the names that you are supposed to know. When we went, everyone comes with a box. Within one week, you show one medicine at a time, so you know what it does and what it treats . . .*

My mother is the one who used to do midwife work. She does it back at home. I was told by my mother, "This is the work you will be doing and it is going to give you food for your children." And it is the work that sustains me. And my grandmother was a midwife . . . My mother still delivers. She even came here.

My mother is the type she eats food that is not cooked with oil. She is still stronger than I am. Even if you see her in this photo, you will be shocked.

Before I traveled to the Continent to interview midwives, I expected that most mothers would still be giving birth outside of hospitals. In the past, midwives in Korogocho had supported and cared for mothers who preferred to give birth outside of the hospital by turning their homes into modified birth centers where a room was set aside for labor and birth. I would later meet another midwife, Elizabeth, who even posted a hand-painted birth center sign in the room where she was once busy assisting mothers during labor and birth. Now, similar to Naomi, Elizabeth has designated that space for providing massages and using her hands to determine when a mother might expect to give birth. "Some come at two months. I look and I just touch, and I can feel if she is pregnant. Then there are those who come for massage," Elizabeth told me. So while fewer women were coming to Elizabeth seeking her services during labor and birth, Elizabeth and Naomi continued to provide massages, advice, and social supports for pregnant women in their community.

Even when planning to have their baby in the hospital, some mothers also continued to count on the skills of midwives like Naomi and Elizabeth to recommend when their labor intensified enough for them to go to the hospital to avoid pharmaceutical interventions sometimes used to intensify contractions during labor. Mothers also counted on the massage techniques of midwives to determine the position of the baby in utero. An infant who presents head first is ideally positioned for a vaginal birth.

Naomi described how she used her hand skills to reposition a baby while still in the womb as a way to prevent complications that might lead to medical interventions such as a caesarean section.

NAOMI: *From my mother, I learned how to check a person. I don't help a person I have not checked to deliver because I don't know how the baby is lying. If the baby is lying in a bad position, I turn it and it becomes okay. As long as I touch you like this, I know how the baby is lying. There is herbal medicine which has been kneaded with oil. That is what I touch with. Yes, God granted me that. There is no problem with that. There is some medicine you are given. It looks like tea leaves. You just put it in a little water; then after it warms, you give it to her. If the baby is lying in a bad position, you turn the baby so the baby lies well . . . I have medicine. I have a store of medicine. In fact, I normally package for people medicine for 200 shillings. It is tea leaves, but it is medicine. You cannot get illnesses. You will be coming to buy. Let me show you the one for the massage. Let me bring it.*

Naomi continued by describing how she cared for more than one generation of birthing mothers in some families and managed emergencies including caring for a mother in an emergency situation who delivered quintuplets on the side of the road.

NAOMI: *Ever since I started midwifery, no one has ever gotten hurt. Even the ones I assisted in delivering, some are married, (laughs) they have grandchildren. There is no problem. God blessed me there. It is not a lie. And I started in '83. There was even one woman who delivered five children. She gave birth to five and I assisted her by the roadside. So I carried her. I was just walking, so I carried her and took her to her house. So two died. They were weak. Three are alive. One is married to my in-law's daughter.*

But it was her skills in massage that Naomi focused on most.

NAOMI: *There are those who come for me to check them, massage them; then they come when it is time to deliver. They start coming at six or five months. And there is a*

*medicine that she is given to take. I touch with my hands
to know.*
    *Many come. Even girls come. Now those who come to
deliver are few. For the young ones, there are those who
don't have children and want to be treated. There are those
who miscarry at two or three months. You just found them
before they were gone.*

As a caregiver, Naomi also respected cultural traditions
that are often dismissed by mainstream providers because they
have yet to be rigorously evaluated by Western science. But in
cultures where the ties between body, mind, and spirit are the
foundation of many spiritually based beliefs, addressing psychological and spiritual concerns is considered as important as
focusing on physical ones during pregnancy, labor, and birth.
For example, midwives in Korogocho recounted how sexual
offenses committed by the father or mother can affect pregnancy and the birthing outcome. Remedies described by the
midwives I met in Korogocho included providing pregnant
mothers instructions on how to prepare herbal baths of purification and protection, for example. In prescribing cleansing practices, midwives in Korogocho described how they are
sometimes guided by their intuition or dreams. In their villages, the midwives I met recalled women also turning to medicine men who were knowledgeable about Luo traditions for
similar prescriptions. Mothers seeking support from midwives
who are respectful of their culturally based traditions persist
even when most mothers now have their babies in hospital.
    In Kenya, medical systems also are finding other ways to
respect culturally based traditions that aim to increase trust in
hospital-based maternity care. At the Ngatataek Hospital in Kaji-
ado, the hospital administration decided to build a traditional
manyatta hut on the hospital grounds to attract mothers who
wanted to continue the ancient tradition of birthing in a familiar village hut surrounded by women they loved and trusted. In

a BBC news clip, "Giving Birth in a Traditional Maasai Hut in Kenya" (December 24, 2018), Yvonne Siano explained that she prefers birthing in a hut because she dislikes the coldness of a delivery room that is overcrowded with hospital staff and prefers the care of a traditional birth attendant (TBA). In the BBC newscast, there is even a clip showing a woman being massaged as Siano explains how "the TBAs take good care of you."

Sarah, the last midwife I interviewed that day, confessed in a whisper that mothers continue to seek her care. Based on her charisma, I could see why she would be a popular provider of birthing care. Even though short in stature, she appeared to be a midwife superstar—reminding me of how I felt when meeting the famed energetic Beninese singer-songwriter Angelique Kujo at the Kennedy Center in Washington, DC. In the heat of the late afternoon, I felt that the spotlight was on Sarah as she came running out to the van to welcome us to the clinic where she now assists with outreach and helps mothers enroll for free prenatal care.

Sarah voiced strength and determination in wanting to continue her midwife practice. Like the other midwives I met that day, her practice included a reliance on her massage techniques. Along with providing massages during pregnancy, Sarah also explained how she relied on her massage techniques to determine the position of the baby throughout the various stages of labor.

While Sarah no longer reserves a room in her house for mothers who choose an out-of-hospital birth, this midwife remains proud of her birthing outcomes and proudly described her skills in caring for mothers who might face challenges when giving birth because the baby may not be in the ideal birthing position. Rather than attribute her success to her own skills, Sarah gave God the credit for her accomplishments in caring for women who presented with unexpected complications.

SARAH: *Yes, even now I am massaging them. Now they are going to the hospital and they found that the baby is sitting down, they come to me from very far, even many come from Kawngware. Some come from Ngong. Some come from Thika. Those who know me because the baby is sitting down come and I turn her baby. She is not operated on. Her baby turns well, and she delivers well. I check the baby before she or he is born. I check so when I have confirmed everything is okay there, that is when I release her.*

Confident in her skills, Sarah remains optimistic about eventually returning to her midwife practice even though she is unable to be certified as a TBA in Nairobi (because of the government's initiative to have all babies born in hospital). Sarah was the only midwife I met, however, who had employed her massage skills in hospital settings in the past. Working in the hospital in a position that was similar to a nurses' aide, Sarah said, "Doctors would call on me to assist in turning the baby even after the mother was in the hospital." Sarah's confidence that her midwifery will continue also stems from her belief that she was spiritually chosen to be a midwife.

> SARAH: *So now if I could get a license, I will do my work. Because as many come here and tell me, "We have passed your house and we did not get you. Why have you removed the beds out of the house?" You can even hear this one asking me where I have taken the beds to. It is a license that I don't have. I started my hospital. I put up my beds. I used to deliver at my house. I had an aunt who was a midwife. I was not taught by my aunt, but it came to me. Let's say it's like I was born with that gift.*

In my first day of interviewing midwives in Kenya, I was given several healing plants, and their stories grounded me in the work of interviewing midwives that I would continue in Kenya, Ethiopia, and Ghana in the ensuing weeks. As I was leaving Korogocho, mothers carrying babies and young children accompanied me back to the van as if I were part of a grand ceremonial parade. "We believe by walking at least half-way down the road with the person leaving, the person will return," the interpreter explained.

During the following days in Nairobi, I began my mornings drinking tea made from these plants that had sprouted up out of the rich and fertile ground, growing toward the light and up through the mounds of plastic and rubbish surrounding the settlement. Drinking the tea felt like a celebration of my return to the Continent, connecting me to my African ancestry and taking me a step closer to my spiritual destiny. It also confirmed that I would be receiving the massage from Naomi that she had gently suggested that I needed.

CHAPTER 2

Baringo County

Naming Traditions, Pouring Libations, Preparing Fermented Milk

After leaving Nairobi, I began a ride into the unknown with Elkanah, the driver of a Speed Link Tours van. Once free of Nairobi's snarling traffic, Elkanah treated me like an American tourist interested in an African safari. I resisted stopping to snap photos on the highway of cargo trucks that linked Nairobi to Mombasa, where the Chinese government was supporting building a new railroad line connecting the two cities. When he suggested stopping on the highway for me to take photos of zebras and chimpanzees, I wanted to explain that I was not a tourist on a safari. Didn't he understand that I was his African sister who had come to the Continent on a homecoming journey to find out the birthing traditions of my ancestors, who could also be his ancestors? But before I could explain about the genealogical work I was doing, I noticed a chimpanzee mom sheltering her newborn just off the highway. So I smiled and said "yes" to taking pictures with my phone.

Three hours later, I checked into Tady's Hotel, described by friends as the best Eldama Ravine offers, just in time for an early supper. As I sensed the waiter was delighted in having a chance to strongly recommend the delicious Kentucky fried chicken to a Black person from the US, I had a hard time convincing him that I really wanted the soup with African vegetables which would become my favorite for breakfast and dinner the four days I was there. I worried that midwives in Eldama Ravine and surrounding Baringo County might see me as an American to impress with the lessons learned from their government-sponsored TBA training programs rather than focusing on naming ceremonies, rituals, and other traditions they had sustained. The next morning at 8 a.m., a health department official welcomed me to Baringo County, and then I headed to a Nubian village in Eldama Ravine to interview midwives.

As early as the 12th century, Nubians from the Sudan began a southern migration into Ethiopia and Kenya. In 1887 the British Empire forced Nubians out of the Sudan to serve in the colonial military and build a railroad. The Sudanese laborers eventually established their own community in Eldama Ravine, a few miles north of the equator.

The first midwife I met in Baringo County was a descendant of the 19th-century Nubians who established Eldama Ravine, the district capital of Baringo County. Wearing a flowing, golden-yellow, ankle-length tunic, Khadijah, 62 years old, welcomed me into her home filled with lace-adorned chairs, tables, and couches. Her brilliant red head covering reflected the strength and dignity of her spirit, which became even more apparent as she described her family's deep roots in Eldama Ravine. Her family lineage includes her grandmother, a midwife who was respected for sustaining traditional birthing rituals. "My family has lived here for years. My grandmother was a TBA and when she decided to stop, I took her place," Khadijah said. "She wanted to give it to my mother, but she was too afraid. My grandmother passed me the knowledge because I wasn't afraid to do the delivery." Khadijah also remembered traditions and rituals that her grandmother respected, including naming ceremonies.

KHADIJAH: *My grandmother would be saying "Bismillah rahman Rahim" starting with the name of the God and calling this child of "this father," quoting the name of the* father. *She would then give the mother some water to drink. When the mother finishes drinking the water, the baby will have come down. Then she also says the name of that day in the week so the child can be named after that day. For instance, if it is Thursday, that child can be named after that day. The baby is named Khamis, meaning Thursday.*

Right after birth the mother is given hot water to drink every now and then and honey and porridge to avoid a stomachache. The mother was protected by the burning fire. That fire was kept warming the house for 24 hours to keep the mother and baby warm inside the house.

Khadijah also explained how her grandmother was recognized at the formal naming ceremony.

KHADIJAH: *The entire village gathered and a goat might be slaughtered. My grandmother might be given the best part of the goat. At the celebration, the infant was then presented with a formal name given to the newborn by a grandmother, if a girl, and a grandfather, if a boy. The name was carefully selected by the grandparents based on communication with the ancestors. It was the ancestor who named the child.*

While Khadijah described a tradition of newborns given a name based on the day they were born, other midwives described how names were determined according to the time of day the mother gave birth. Born in Kabartonjo, Kenya, in 1960, Rachael practiced as a midwife in the mountainous region of Lembus in the village of Kipkanyilat. The forests of Lembus once shielded the Mau Mau people and provided a hideaway for Jomo Kenyatta, who became the first president of the newly independent Kenya in 1960.

Along with learning her midwifery skills from her mother, Tortok, Rachael was also knowledgeable about other practices to promote well-being in body, mind, and spirit during pregnancy and birth, such as using massage to determine the position of the baby in utero and avoiding the eating of meat and certain fruits. The eating of ground-up white or red clay stones was also a common practice. I seldom asked midwives to provide a justification for practices recommended to them by elders in the community. For the most part, the women I interviewed accepted without qualifiers the wisdom of grandmothers who knew clays that stored nutrients.

In the village of Kabartonjo, there were also rituals that had a role in making certain that the mother's psychological and spiritual well-being were optimal at the time of birth. Similar to the midwives in Korogocho, Rachael explained that when a sexual offense has been committed by the mother or the father, the midwife recommends herbal baths of purification for the mother as well as the offender making a formal request for forgiveness. Even in the midst of labor, a midwife might summon the offender to the birthing space to apologize. Considered a blessing for the mother, this apology sometimes included the tradition of spitting known as *sere*. The Maasai also view spitting into their palms before shaking hands as a blessing or a way to show endorsement of another person. When used in this way, saliva was viewed as a bodily fluid that had the power to symbolize not only a bodily cleansing but also spiritual purification.

Rachael also described a postpartum ceremony known as "eating the tail," wherein once the umbilical cord was cut, the women who had supported the mother through labor and birth would gather for food and drinking of tea. In a celebratory ritual following the birth, the meal included the so-called eating of the tail. This midwife was told by elders as a child that "eating the tail" was a metaphor rather than what that I thought might be, the physical eating of the umbilical cord which had nourished the newborn infant while still in the womb (a practice that is regaining some popularity due to the umbilical cord being the source of nutrition for the infant prior to birth). Instead,

Rachael believed that the phrase meant the eating of a particular food and was a way of indicating that after the cord was cut, the child's spirit would live in them. The ritual reminded me in some ways of the symbolism of eating the blessed parcel of bread served at communion.

Like other midwives in Baringo County, Rachael was a lineage midwife. Her mother was recognized and respected as a midwife in Kabartonjo prior to Rachael accepting the role as midwife in her community.

RACHAEL: I learned from my mother. When she was close, she would call me to help her fetch some things. I respected the older midwives because they respected the mothers . . .

If the baby was born at night around 8 p.m. to 9 p.m., they would name the baby Kiplagat [a boy] or Chelagat [a girl]; if born at midnight or around 2 a.m., the child would be named Kipkemoi [a boy] or Chekemoi [a girl]; if born in the morning, the child is named Kimutai [a boy] or Chemutai [a girl]; in the daytime, Kibet [a boy], or for the girl, Chebet. It all depended on the time. Then came the singing of songs with the child's name. The midwives chose the names of infants, and that name was then given to the clinic to be placed on the birthing certificate . . .

Long time ago when a child was born, those midwives the age of my mother would congregate themselves where the child was born and claim they are eating the child's tail; then they celebrate. It involved cooking Ugali and gifting those who are there and naming the child, but these days, we don't do that practice anymore . . .

Sarah, born in northern Baringo County in 1959 and also immersed in the ways of her grandmother, described the extent to which she respected the traditions followed by the grandmothers who had not converted to Christianity or Islam but who continued to call on "Cheptalel," a traditional Kenyan name for God. Ethnic groups who refer to God as Cheptalel in Kenya mostly settled in communities in the northern part of Kenya and may refer to Cheptalel as masculine or feminine. Traditions included keeping the fire burning at birth for several months.

SARAH: *I learned from a woman older than me. When she was called to help, she would ask me to go with her. My friends are old. I love spending time with older people. I think she saw that I am a person who likes listening to advice from the old women. Those times people didn't go to hospitals, so whenever they were called upon to help the other deliver, they would ask me to come to see how they did it . . .*

They used fire for lighting, and they would ask me to make a fire so they could see clearly. I used to see the mother sit properly on a stone. The mothers should stay steady . . .

After the birth we clean the birthplace and place the mother on the bed. Then they give the child the family name and later a religious name. You don't give a name belonging to someone who used to be very angry most of the time; you give the name of a person who has a good character.

They would prepare dry firewood and let the mother light the fire and then ensure that the fire does not go out. The mother stayed inside for three months. The husband or someone else helped her to cook . . .

When I was helping the mothers, I wasn't saved. I just asked the Cheptalel, "May God look after woman." We were not afraid.

In olden times they called the midwife "Jorwab Kawa," meaning a friend of the child. They used to respect the midwives, and after the child has grown, they come to the midwives and look for her and also bring a gift—honey, millet—or just go and feed them. I used to love it, and I also have a heart of loving. I love being called a friend to many.

All the younger midwives I met in Baringo County recognized their grandmothers, a mother-in-law, or a mother as the wisdom keeper they apprenticed with and who infused the birth experience with spiritual meaning. "My mother-in-law was a midwife," Makena, another midwife I spoke with, explained. "I stayed with her through all the years of my giving birth," she said with pride.

Makena described how her mother-in-law cared for her during pregnancy using grease to massage her stomach and to determine the position of the baby, and natural medicines and herbs to heal stomach pain. The birthing ceremonies Makena described are similar to those described by other midwives in Baringo County, which included respecting naming traditions and calling on the ancestors.

MAKENA: *I decided to be a midwife on my own after my mother-in-law was old, around [the] late '70s. When a mother was in labor, she would help to give birth and also help in the whole process . . . And the mother would sit on a stone and another one would squat to receive the baby . . . When the child is born in the evening, the baby is named Kiprono or Cherono, and in the morning, Chepkoech or Kipkoech. If the child is a boy, it's the role of [the] father to name the baby, and if it's a girl it is the role of the mother. Later they get another name when the baby's older. The names may be of other relatives who died. They would just gaze into the fire, and at times they would call them after that person. My mother-in-law would speak to the ancestors while spilling milk. She also would do that when a child was sick or a mother was having difficulty. She would call upon the ancestors to come. She would say,*

"We give you this child." Nowadays we pray to God, but in olden days, we would also pray to the ancestors.

Baringo County, which once protected the Mau Mau warriors who succeeded in overturning colonial rule, also sheltered birthing traditions as long as pregnant women did not have any transportation other than a bicycle to travel long distances on often bumpy dirt roads to have their babies in a hospital.

Makena also described libations as part of the birthing ceremony. The spilling of milk is a ceremonial practice not only in some birthing rituals but also in sealing agreements and marking significant rites of passage, such as initiations, weddings, and stepping down from a position as warrior to become an elder, and is a cultural trait found among ethnic groups in Kenya.

Makena explained that birthing traditions supported by her mother-in-law, whom families gifted with blankets or sometimes a jacket rather than cash, are not continued by her. About the traditional practices she described, Makena said, "I left doing those things. Life has improved so we left using stones and bought new stools and learned from the hospital." Specifically, Makena explained the practices she chose to continue and those she abandoned. "So, I stopped making them sit on stones and made them lie down and only one person can assist. I also left child naming to mothers." Yet in other ways Makena still values her mother-in-law's influence on her practice as a midwife: "The most important thing I learned from her is good character and how to work hard and how to care for the children."

Makena also valued the training she is receiving now as a TBA. According to a recent Baringo County campaign to reduce the staggeringly high infant mortality rates in the county, the solution is providing access to free medical care at hospitals and maternity centers in addition to building better roads. But as head of the Office of Minority Health in the New Jersey Department of Health and Senior Services in the US, I learned firsthand that ongoing health disparities persist despite increasing access to hospital-based obstetric care.

Unfortunately, the Baringo County campaign makes no mention of how traditional midwives continue to be respected for their skills and their support of birthing mothers. The campaign also overlooks younger TBAs who enroll in training programs patterned after historical Western-based medical models that have failed to create equity in birthing outcomes. Baringo County has succeeded in improving outcomes for high-risk mothers for whom medical care was previously inaccessible. Unfortunately, their campaign also ignores the successes of traditional midwives in providing successful, compassionate, and culturally sensitive care for mothers even when they present with complications.

Several of the midwives like Makena whom I met in Baringo County described themselves as newly trained TBAs, but Kamia—like Khadijah, the first midwife I met—was different in how she proudly carried her seniority as an elder. Thousands of feet above sea level and a short distance from the equator, I visited a small village of traditional grass huts where respect for Kamia, a traditional senior village midwife, was palpable. It was the day of the spring equinox, and unlike the other midwives I had met, Kamia was not there when I arrived with the translator. We waited more than an hour for Kamia to return to the village, which gave me welcomed time to play with children, hold babies, and spend time in a grass hut for the first time. I could easily imagine staring into the open pit that held the fire, known as the birth fire, that not only provided light but was a source of spiritual protection while waiting for an infant to come into the world and for an ancestral spirit to descend as the midwife provided an appropriate name based on how much light was visible in the sky.

As Kamia approached, the adults and children gathered at the edge of the village, standing in respect to watch Kamia walk up the road with her cow. Long before Kamia's arrival, we knew that the respected elder and midwife was on her way from verbal messages sent ahead by passersby. Wearing a brilliant red dress with splashes of white complementing her powerful charcoal skin tones, Kamia arrived like royalty and then easily positioned herself squatting down to seat herself on a bench close to the ground. Like others I interviewed, Kamia began her story by proudly describing how she was a midwife descendant. "My grandmother chose me," Kamia said, explaining how her grandmother, a midwife, chose her to learn the ways of midwifery practice. Although Kamia said she had no idea of her age, she knew she had delivered 39 babies.

From her grandmother, Kamia explained, she learned how to use a naturally made grease to massage a pregnant mother's stomach and to determine the position of the baby. And this midwife also later followed her grandmother's advice of recommending that mothers eat porridge made from millet flour to give them the strength and energy needed for birthing. For mothers anxious about their pregnancy, Kamia recommended herbal baths and making tea from *chebirirbeiyee,* an herbal medicine. From her grandmother, Kamia learned how to stand behind the mother as she pushed out the baby and how to cut the umbilical cord. This was the only midwife I met who remembered her grandmother cutting the cord with an arrow that she always carried with her to births. Kamia also learned how to cut the cord with an arrow. A woman proudly walking through the village with her arrow as a symbol of her skills may have evoked the kind of respect for a woman that was similar to that afforded a man.

"My grandmother was not given payment. She was given tea or local brew," Kamia explained, looking down at the infant she held in her arms. "She was recognized. She was loved."

Even so, Kamia quickly added, "I have changed now to be a modern woman." Before our conversation ended, I asked Kamia whether she thought anything she learned from her grandmother should be passed on to doctors practicing today. "No. I can't tell certain things to young people because of their age,"

Kamia said, gently rocking one of her young grandchildren in her arms.

Walking back through a gate made out of tree branches, I noticed the gate appeared to be structured so that it would never close (see figure 2.1). As dust seeped into my sandals, I began to believe that the birthing stories I heard in Baringo County were told like biblical stories with old and new testaments.

As I walked through the open gate, at the edge of Kamia's family village, I felt on top of the world and graced by the presence of Cheptalel, God called by a feminine name, as one of the midwives I interviewed in Baringo County explained. At that moment, I sensed Cheptalel's spirit sweeping through the branches of trees on the mountaintop that appeared to be touched by low-hanging clouds. That's when I remembered that it was the spring equinox.

Once back in the van, I thought about Kamia explaining how only elders know about certain traditions related to birthing. I realized then that I will never know how much Kamia left out of the birthing stories that she shared with me because I am not a part of her village or an elder.

A tradition widely supported by midwives in Baringo County that Kamia did not mention in a conversation that seemed more filled with attentiveness and love than information is that reserving *mursik*—traditional fermented milk—in a decorated gourd for the mother to drink at the time of birth is also widely supported by midwives. In the house of a pregnant woman, the mursik-filled gourd is placed on a table or in a visible spot so that everyone entering the house knows that the woman of the house will soon be giving birth (see figure 2.2). The drinking of mursik is recommended by traditional midwives and by contemporary nutritionists. Nutritionists recommend mursik to pregnant mothers because it is higher in protein then fresh milk, and it is easier to digest for Africans, who have a higher incidence of lactose intolerance. Mothers in Baringo County teach their daughters at an early age how to prepare the milk to be

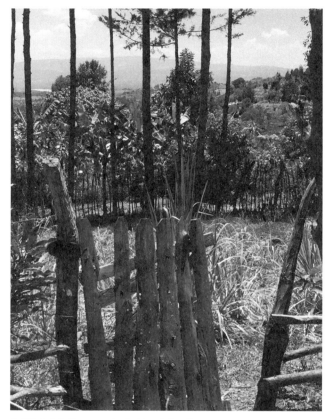

FIGURE 2.1. Open gate in Kamia's village

stored in a decorated gourd (after it is lined with the soot of charcoal made from specific medicinal trees such as the *uset* tree, known for its healing properties).

In Baringo County, a midwife's family provided me lessons in how to make and preserve mursik. The process began with cheering on the young boy who adeptly climbed a tree with amazing speed to select the ideal branch for stirring the fresh cow's milk. Then women passed the selected branch through the fire to coat it with charcoal made from the uset tree. The stirring of the mursik in the gourd reminded me of gentle rhythmic dancing. Women explained that young girls are taught the

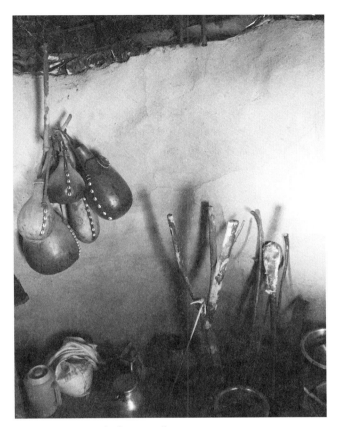

FIGURE 2.2. Gourds for mursik

making of mursik before they are married. When I was passed the stick to practice the stirring, the women laughed at my awkwardness and lack of skill. I joined the laughter as I explained, "I've never been married."

Preparing to leave Baringo County the day after meeting Kamia, I thought about Khadijah, the first midwife I met in this place of breathtaking beauty. Like the last interview, the first interview lingered with me. After our interview, Khadijah held her hands open and nodded for me to place each of my hands on top of her palms. As she firmly grasped my hands, I believed that our spirits connected, and I knew by the force of her grip that our bond would withstand separation. Surely that's how mothers felt when they left the house of their grandmothers, midwives who not only supported them throughout labor and birth but cared for them and fed them for the three days following birth.

On the highway going back to Nairobi, rather than looking out the Speedy Tour van window for wildlife on the side of the road to photograph, I closed my eyes and entered a timeless space as I listened to the chanting of a midwife who surprised me by letting me record her. Several midwives explained that at the time of birth, chanting surrounded the birthing experience. That's when I remembered how Alabama midwives had told me decades ago that while patiently waiting for a baby "to get born," they would fill the room with a hum.

CHAPTER 3

Wolaita Sodo

Caretakers of the Process

After ten days in Kenya, I boarded Ethiopian Airlines, founded in 1945 and the first to be owned by an African nation. Arriving in Addis Ababa, I relaxed into my Blackness, feeling protected and free, having landed in the only nation on the African continent that has never been colonized. Ethiopia is the only place where young school-aged girls ran up to me, touched my skin, and then pointed to their hands and emphatically proclaimed "Black!" as if it was the most important word in their vocabulary.

My time in Ethiopia began with interviewing traditional midwives in Wolaita Sodo, the administrative capital and one of the nine districts in the Southern Nations, Nationalities, and Peoples' Region of Ethiopia. Travel from Addis to Wolaita Sodo required taking an hour-long flight to Arba Minch, followed by a two-hour jeep ride through lush mountains that opened up into stretches of trees abundant with mangos, papayas, and bananas like a Garden of Eden, on land that is now mostly owned by multinational corporations.

Wolaita is translated as "to come together." More than a hundred diverse clans make up the region that flourished for centuries as the independent Wolaita Kingdom until being defeated by the Abyssinian North in the 19th century. More recently, the Wolaita Sodo region challenged government mandates that legislated that it abandon its ancient Afro-Asiatic-based Wolaytta language and adopt Aroma, the official language of northern Ethiopia. Those government mandates failed. That spirit of resistance persists among the midwives I met in the region, who continue to serve as caretakers of ancient birthing traditions and to support women in holistic ways that focus on meeting not only physical but also spiritual and emotional needs. Though government mandates increasingly require mothers to move away from midwife-supported home birth and restrict government support of birthing care to maternity care facilities or hospitals, the traditional midwives and mothers I met in Wolaita Sodo are resisting. They continue to focus on ways of caring that respect traditions and provide emotional support during pregnancy and birth. Massage, touch, ceremonies, rituals, healing herbs, and prayers that promote peace of mind, relaxation, and self-confidence are at the center of these midwives' timeless ways of caring.

Wearing an ankle-length, traditional Ethiopian snow-white dress with an embroidered belt that weaved together threads of orange and green around her waist, Utalo Una, the first midwife I met in Kembata, suggested sitting under a tree that appeared to be the central gathering place in her village. As we watched school-aged boys a few feet away play an old-time game of stickball that involves rolling a tire with a stick, our conversation began with Una describing her path to becoming a midwife. Una also explained how mothers chose her as a midwife because they knew her to be a compassionate caregiver.

> UNA: *My name is Utalo Una. I don't know my age, but it could be 50 years. I was born here in my village called Wachiga. There was my uncle's wife [my aunt] during Emperor Haile Silassie's regime who was a TBA. She passed away long years ago . . .*
>
> *There was one neighborhood TBA who encouraged me to be engaged in supporting a woman who is in labor. And*

most of my families and neighbors recommended me, saying, "You are kind enough, compassionate, and a respectful mother, so you better support us . . ." Initially I was very fearful to be left alone conducting a delivery or even observing a mother who is in labor. With God's support, I'm [still] very successful today in my career as a TBA. The community values, respects, and trusts us. That is our source of satisfaction.

When describing her midwifery skills, Una focused on massage as a central part of her practice. While proud of her technique in determining the baby's position in the womb, Una also valued learning how to provide a sensitive and comforting massage from the way her birth attendant cared for her.

UNA: *My birth attendant provided me a light touch without pressuring the womb to facilitate the labor progress. Doing so, she could identify the position of the baby in the womb. While providing a massage all over the body as needed, I also can find any sign of pain . . . I would give the massage before birth and during labor to help keep the baby in the correct position. The massage is also very important to identify whether the mother is pregnant with twins or not, because the TBAs do not have any medical equipment for that situation. After birth, I continue with the massage until the placenta is released. I also massage the newborn after cutting the cord so that the infant does not end up having an extended stomach . . . I don't believe that the health care workers are able to practice the massage that we do for easing labor . . . For the massage I use an oil or butter to avoid a rough touch and to correct the position of the baby, if needed.*

Continuing to emphasize the importance of relaxation, Una described how she turned to her garden for herbs that reduced tensions and prevented more stressful operative procedures, such as caesarean sections. When I asked about herbs, Una immediately pointed to her garden a few feet away and asked a man—who proudly stood nearby, nodding in agreement with Una's comments—to pull a specific herb from the corner of the garden (see figure 3.1); this herb she pounded down to make teas that provided strength during pregnancy and eased pain during childbirth. She also used homegrown spices to prepare drinks that helped open the cervix and shorten labor. Showing the depth of her herbal knowledge, Una explained how she used another plant to make a tea that is effective in avoiding the operative procedures that "are happening more and more in the maternity facilities." When caring for a mother who may be emotionally stressed, Una pointed out two different plants in her garden of pharmacopeia that she mixed with butter to help ease labor pains and promote relaxation.

While Una had an established fee for her services, she did not see payment as a reward for her personal success in "delivering" a baby. For Una, the birth of a healthy baby is a gift from the Creator. Una even viewed making pronouncements about her success (including keeping count of the babies and mothers she successfully cared for) as inappropriate. Una saw her humility as contributing to her ability to invest her energy in focusing on the well-being of the mother and baby instead of on reward or honor from the mother or the community she served.

> UNA: *Sometimes I was paid 20 to 100 ETBs [58 cents to 3 US dollars]. Other times, they just will share a coffee at the end . . . I don't know how many babies I have delivered, since I have been doing this for decades. Also, counting the numbers is a sin for me. God dislikes it. I don't want to talk further about this issue. God does not like us counting babies. It is a sin.*

Other midwives I met in Wolaita Sodo also credited God for their success. For example, although Simo Tembebo, a midwife who lived in the Kembata District of Wolaita Sodo, credited her

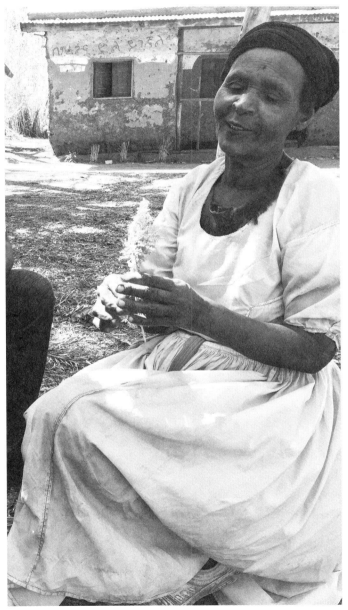

FIGURE 3.1. Midwife Utalo Una holding an herb in Kembata, Wolaita Sodo

mother with preparing her with the skills needed to become a skillful and caring midwife, she also credits her constant communication with God as the foundation of her success. Before attending a birth, Tembebo turns to prayer as a way to humble herself and recognize God's power and strength. Tembebo also enters the birthing space with a mindset of humility and focuses on caring rather than directing or controlling the birth experience. Reflecting ancient African traditional religions that honor spirits that live in nature, rivers, and all living creatures including animals, Tembebo's prayers connect with the spiritual practices and beliefs of mothers who continue to honor the ways of their mothers and grandmothers who were the traditional caregivers in their pastoral communities.

TEMBEBO: *I do pray by kneeling down to God for an hour. Without prayer, I do nothing. These are my words: "God, you're the one whose bones and flesh created a man in a woman's womb. Also, you are the one who made the lamb in a sheep's womb and a calf in a cow's womb. If you are willing, please give us this child without any trouble as you made it in the womb. Kindly help us to help this child." And these are the words we use.*

Before becoming a midwife, Tembebo learned her ways of serving childbearing women through an apprenticeship with her mother, who was also known as a caring and respected "mother" to many women in her village and beyond.

TEMBEBO: *My mother was known as a TBA from my childhood. I used to follow my mother when she would go to attend a birth because people came from different directions looking for my mother's help. She had great respect from the community. Then, everyone called the midwife "Mother." Now they call midwives "doctors" . . . Before, people used to come to me from different areas, even on horses, looking for me for help, and I was working inde-*

pendently, but now the government forces every mother to give birth at health facilities. The laboring mother prefers home because health facilities or hospitals are too cold, but at home, they say they get enough heat and care.

Homebirth with a midwife also offered the advantage of being prescribed the same familiar foods and teas that their mothers or grandmothers had prescribed. Tembebo and other midwives suggested eating porridges made from local grains for strength during pregnancy and in the early stages of labor. Because the foods were familiar and easy to get in the open market, recommendations from midwives, like eating extra doses of the Ethiopian banana, enset, or the "false banana," were also easy to follow.

> TEMBEBO: *I recommend that mothers prepare a variety of foods . . . I used to give herbal medicine to pregnant women, but now the government has taught us to not give such things, but I do tell pregnant woman to eat vegetables, porridge, and oats four to five times per day. If not, you will become weak.*
>
> *I tell them to prepare porridge from flour prepared from various cereals such as bean, sorghum, and porridge from the local banana [enset]. It helps strengthen both the mother and fetus because it is prepared with butter.*

In addition to its use in both massage and for nutrition, butter has symbolic significance in Wolaita Sodo because of the way it is used in traditional ceremonies and blessing rituals. For example, many regional rituals involve the bride covering her skin with butter mixed with clay for an extended period before the beginning of the wedding ceremony. In ancient times in the kingdom of Wolaita Sodo, warriors painted their chest with red soil mixed with butter before going into battle, and women honored heroic warriors when they returned by spontaneously spilling butter over their heads when meeting them in the marketplace. A midwife who drenched a mother's body with butter for massage during labor was using an oil that symbolized protection and respect.

In a heavily trafficked community center in the town of Wolaita Sodo, the administrative center of the Wolaita Zone, there is a prominent monument of a man and woman embracing as one and drinking butter from a shared vessel. The monument is a symbol of how Wolaita Sodo unites a culturally diverse region of two million people that includes a large number of pastoral farmers through the ceremonious drinking of butter. Behind the monument is a powerful image of the revered Ka wo [King] Tona, the last king of the Wolaita Kingdom before they were defeated by the Abyssinian Army of Northern Ethiopia.

While rituals associated with the drinking of butter provide energy for the mother during the birthing process, the coffee ceremonies that follow birth create a space for strengthening bonds, reciting prayers, sharing stories, remembering the past, welcoming, laughing, and showing other ways of caring. Tembebo described how following the birth, a coffee ceremony is when women share the joy of birth. "A hot drink for the baby's mother will be given and a coffee ceremony will be prepared," Tembebo explained. "The neighbors bring coffee and other food and drinks for the neighboring mothers and relatives who come to celebrate."

Ayelech Hafamo, the only midwife I met while in Wolaita Sodo who provided details about receiving formal TBA training, supports upholding cultural traditions along with valuing her formal training for being an active midwife focused on assessing the mother and infant for problems and risks.

> HAFAMO: Yes, we do shout and dance. We do drink and eat while the mother holds and breastfeeds the baby. The neighboring mothers and the mother of the husband must be there if she is alive. I name the baby based on the season or [on whether] it is day or night. Sometimes the family of the newborn gives the name according to their will and

reasons. I may do it the first time at the birth place, but the family changes the name sometimes.

Regarding her midwifery skills, Hafamo described her three months of formal midwife training when she was forced to live in a relocation camp in Northwest Ethiopia. Now, decades after becoming a midwife who once attended as many as ten babies in one day, Hafamo no longer uses her skills as an experienced midwife. Now Hafamo is concerned about the lack of emotional support mothers receive when giving birth in a hospital setting or maternity facility where practitioners often don't consider the mother's feelings as part of their care.

HAFAMO: *I was born at Wadole [South Ethiopia, along road of Hossana to Wolaita Sodo]*
I don't know exactly when, but as I heard it from my family, it may have been around the 1950s or '60s.
I was taken by the government to a relocation program [in the] Gambella [Northwest Ethiopia] region, and there I received three months of training by white women to prepare me for being a TBA. The trainers gave us bowls to hold soap, and a dish, so we can boil the blade, and we were given bags to hold the material that helped me to help the mothers. I used to go to pregnant women in order to check how they feel and what they are eating. Every day I went to the health facilities to visit and assist pregnant and laboring mothers there. I got a lot of certificates of accomplishment. Then the war came, and we were relocated. Because of unrest, I left and came back to my homeland with my two kids. When I left, I left every certificate that tells of my experience and the material I used except for a bowl that I used to hold soap and the dish I used when I boiled the blade. Three years later, one woman who knew about my experience as a TBA came from Gambella and gave information to the health center. Then the health center confirmed my experience, and I continued as a TBA . . .

I do have experience determining [whether] there is problem in the position or the presentation. If I feel the position seems not right, I try to correct that through massage. If I can't, I tell the relatives to take her to the hospital by preparing the transportation. As the time of labor approaches, I tell the woman to prepare porridge and oats of a mixture of various cereals. Bleeding sometimes occurs before the mother gives birth. If this happens, I quickly take the woman to the hospital. But after she has given birth, I wait for ten minutes observing for bleeding. I do recommend food that helps stop bleeding by cleaning out what remains by giving her palm oats to drink.

Hafamo explained that because the government is now against home delivery, she only checks pregnant women when a mother comes to her to see whether they are close to the time of giving birth. After checking them, Hafamo said, "I send them to health facilities where they can get skilled birth attendants." Hafamo, however, not only remains confident in her skills; she is also convinced that if traditional midwives like herself were allowed to continue their practice, they could reduce escalating caesarean section rates. Hafamo argued that her skills in positioning the baby in utero through massage would have an impact in reducing the need to sedate mothers for invasive surgical procedures. The cold and sterile environments of delivery rooms are also a cause of stress and anxiety; mothers previously gave birth in environments where women committed themselves to keep fires burning and they could feel the warmth of their collective presence.

HAFAMO: *I asked the government to let us participate in the health facilities to share our knowledge to prevent a lot of unnecessary caesarean sections and deaths that occur in the hospitals. It is unfair. The community still looks for our help.*

They refuse us because they believe they are profes-
sional and follow scientific principles. It is unfair for them
just to ignore us. I asked the government to let us practice
to reduce caesarean sections.

When scholars at the University of Wolaita Sodo conducted a 2018 survey, they found that mothers had similar concerns about birthing in maternity care facilities and hospitals. The researchers documented rampant complaints about being disrespected and even reported that women complained of receiving inhumane treatment that included abuse. The women provided specific examples of a lack of cultural acceptance and respect for the traditions they valued. For example, nursing staff refused to let them take the afterbirth home for proper burial. There was also a problem of a lack of emotional support, as one mother complained: "No one cares for our feelings."

Four days after arriving in Wolaita Sodo, I boarded a crowded bus before dawn on a Sunday morning to head back to Arba Minch to catch a returning flight to Addis. When suddenly awakened by the wailing of an elderly woman sitting across the aisle from me on the bus, I thought she might be ill. The passenger next to me explained, "They are saying that her brother died, and she is going to his funeral in Arba Minch. Because we are getting close to Arba Minch, she is overcome with grief."

The chatter on the bus came to a sudden stop as the driver pulled over to the side of the road and parked the bus. The fierce-sounding man who earlier stood in the aisle making sure everyone was in their assigned seats, collected tickets without any greetings, and barked at passengers for not securing their suitcases on the overhead rack suddenly transformed himself into a compassionate caregiver. As silence fell over the bus, the bus operator slowly walked up the aisle to the back of the bus and sat down in the vacated seat next to the wailing woman. He held her hand and cared for her feelings, and I was struck by the similarity in care to the ways of a traditional midwife.

CHAPTER 4

Afar

Timeless Bonds, Smoking the Mother, Extended Care

Leaving the lush greenery of Wolaita Sodo to interview midwives in Afar, Ethiopia, I was less than 200 miles from the Danakil Depression, one of the hottest places on Earth; some have described going to the Danakil Depression as a way to experience life on another planet. It was the extreme opposite of the lushness of Wolaita Sodo. But, in Afar, I felt like I had returned to the beginning of time.

Shortly after arriving in Afar's Semera Airport, a 55-minute flight from Addis, I learned that a museum is being built a short distance from the airport that will be the resting place for the 3.5-million-year-old fossilized bones of Dinkinesh (Amharic for "you are marvelous"). European archeologists who listened endlessly to the Beatles' popular song "Lucy in the Sky with Diamonds" during the 1974 dig named her bones "Lucy" in remembrance of the song. After landing in Afar, I stepped onto the arid ground where Dinkinesh once walked.

Historically known for having the largest livestock population in Africa, the Afar region has been occupied by Ethiopian pastoralists, herders, and nomads dating back as far as written and oral records can attest. I began learning my first day in Afar that midwives express a nomadic spirit in their willingness to travel long distances to assist birthing mothers.

Birthing culture in Afar is influenced by the predominance of Muslim, mostly Sunni, religious practices that intermingle with traditions rooted in ancient African spiritual beliefs and rituals. Typically known as *una tilas* [translated as "mothers of the one," the one being the birthing mother], traditional midwives in Afar sustained traditions similar to other practices rooted in African cultures throughout the Continent. The major concern of traditional midwives that I met in Afar is making certain to continue the custom of women receiving emotional, psychological, and spiritual support for an extended period before, during, and after birth, as was the way of their mothers and grandmothers.

Just hours after landing in Sameera, I met two midwives—Hawa Galale Elissa, 30 years old, and Hasna Mohammed Hassen, a 44-year-old midwife. In her desert environment, Hawa called birth "a time between life and death," a way of expressing how fragile life can be for mothers and babies in the days immediately following birth. Despite reports that show progress made in reducing infant and maternal mortality rates, challenges remain. Campaigns to improve outcomes often make increasing access to hospital-based services following Western medical care models the primary focus and overlook root causes that affect birthing outcomes, such as poverty, access to nutritious food, and barriers women face in pursuing educational opportunities. Women I met on the Continent continued to value the social supports that were part of traditional midwifery models for birthing care, describing how women gathered and supported mothers with prayers throughout labor and birth and how the midwife positioned herself closest to the mother and remained by her side not only during birth but in the months that followed.

> HAWA: *In those times in the past, we were not living the way we are living now. We used to live in a scattered way—a house here, another house very far away. The TBA would stay 14–15 days, 20 days, and not go far from me*

until the delivery comes. We kept her nearby our house, giving her all the things she needs. Sometimes they rubbed the body down with leaves made by a traditional healer or they made a tea from the fatty part of the goat's tail.

Mothers stayed outside saying prayers. They didn't come too close because they would feel the pain. Hearing their prayers helped me to take the pain. I could hear the mothers outside saying "May God separate her safely. May God help her in separating peacefully." That is the prayer everyone was saying. The midwife sat beside us.

When Hasna joined the conversation, she explained how she occasionally still practices as a midwife and spoke about what she learned from her mother, who was also a midwife.

HASNA: *I was 15 years old. I was staying at home and a pregnant woman about to deliver came to me and asked me to assist her as I was alone, and she took the risk asking me to do it. I immediately recalled how my mother helped mothers to deliver in the nearby houses. [After that], I became a TBA.*

I learned many good things from my mother—respect people and be serious with my life.

I do know how to stop bleeding during delivery by using traditional leaves, called warabe kala and Atuki, which come from the neighboring districts. These leaves are cleaned and washed and boiled with water to make [something] like tea to drink.

Butter and the fatty part of [a] sheep tail are given to the pregnant mother to make her stronger.

I am still helping in the community when [a] baby's coming is urgent. Otherwise, I go with them to the hospital or health center. The last time I assisted with [a] delivery was two months ago.

What the hospitals and facilities can learn from my mother is [that] our midwives used to travel long distances

*and stayed with pregnant women for weeks to assist moth-
ers who are delivering. Maybe this can still be experienced.*

Midwives in Afar believe that the tradition of providing
extended support and care beyond the time of birthing should
continue even when a woman is giving birth in a health facility or hospital. Momina Abdalla Mussa, 60 years old, who
grew up in the village of Bayahele and now lives in the Dubti
district, emphasized lessons learned from the practices of the
grandmothers who once were the primary source of birthing
care. What mattered most to Momina was extending current
hospital-based birthing practices to include addressing basic
survival needs, such as having enough to eat. Timeless postpartum traditions and feasting celebrations when birthing in the
village, including making certain that special servings of food
are set aside for the mother, are sacrificed when the birthing
takes place long distances from home.

Although the practice of female circumcision is no longer
as ubiquitous as it once was, several midwives in Afar said that
they had been circumcised. Others witnessed their mothers
performing circumcisions and episiotomies that required using
a special knife designated for that purpose. In the Afar warrior
culture, men once gained respect for skillful use of the knife
that made them masters of self-defense. Now, however, the jila,
a treasured knife once used in warfare by men, is mostly worn
for ceremonial purposes, such as when attending intergenera-
tional rituals celebrating newborn babies. Before campaigns to
eliminate the practice of genital mutilation, people also saw the
knife being carried by a midwife as a symbol of her respected
power.

While none of the midwives that I met are supporting campaigns to end female circumcision, they are sympathetic to and
supportive of mothers who are only comfortable with female
caregivers at the time of birth and are insulted and feel deeply
disrespected when men touch intimate parts of their bodies
during examination. Momina described her personal experi-

ence in becoming a midwife and the spiritual and culturally based practices she uses to aid women's pregnancy, labor, and birth. For example, Momina was familiar with geophagy, strong urges to eat selected clays that may have medicinal value during pregnancy. As a midwife, Momina advocated for women who wanted health care facilities to respect religious and culturally based preferences.

MOMINA: *I became a traditional birth attendant by accident one day. I was alone, and a woman came to my house and told me to assist her. I was a little scared, and she told me not to worry and that I had to help her. While I was looking for the Makkita [knife] and could not find it, she told me to use the blade she gave me. I immediately recalled how my mother was doing this in those old days, as I was not taught by her, but I use[d] to see when my mother was doing this nearby our house, so I learned how to position for opening the female organ for removing the baby. I assisted the mother and she delivered safely. That was my first time assisting. After that, everybody came to know me and started calling me Ula Tina [Mother of the One].*

When a woman becomes pregnant, they usually call me when there is an indication that the time for delivery is soon. That's when I shift my place to be nearby the pregnant woman's house to see her closely and follow her.

If a pregnant woman gets sick, there are traditional healers who make Qur'ran verses which are called Pregnancy Papers that are tied on their arms and neck. There are specific verses, but I don't know them. They also may slaughter a goat and tell the mother to eat the liver.

There are some herbal drugs for pain called Damaho. I have it at home, and I can bring it for you to see. Some women during the beginning of pregnancy used to eat a black clay, not here in Dubti, but a little far from here in my village called Beyahele. Here in Dubti there is no black clay that I can see . . .

> When they call me for assistance, I just go and volun-
> teer and I don't get absent because of bad dreams or any-
> thing. What I go for is to assist only. I usually don't charge
> for service. What they send me is part of the goat, Hakele
> [ribs of the goat], which is specifically given for the TBA.
> Now we assist at home only if there is an urgent need.
> We work with health facilities for mothers to deliver
> because they get every intervention needed there. Finally,
> we suggest that we need to be assisted by women and [that]
> the facilities should be ready to prepare food for women
> coming from far places and having no money.

I nodded in agreement as I watched Momina and the other TBAs who had gathered join together in a circle. Moments later, Momina asked me to hand her the white scarf wrapped around my shoulders that I had grabbed from a sale rack in the Whole Foods Market months ago. Momina transformed this everyday cotton scarf into a holy veil to cover my head and some of my face. "We have a new name for you," Momina said, with the grace of a priestess. "We have decided on the name Fateema."

The next day, on the drive to Megenta to interview mid-wives, I realized that the way I received my name reminded me of an impromptu African naming ceremony. I also realized that I had been making assumptions about women who veiled their faces and chose to cover themselves in black robes, which reminded me of Catholic nuns. In the hotel restaurant, I was angered every morning that I never saw a woman in the restaurant unaccompanied by a man, as if I had missed an unwritten sign that made it illegal for a woman to eat alone. The stereotypes in my head were broken when I met the free-spirited, independent, and creative midwives who spontaneously decided to gift me with an Islamic name in a health administrator's office.

The region our jeep traveled through to reach the Megenta health facility contains the most complete hominin record of an environmental setting of human evolution from six million years ago. The dusty road took on ancient reverberations as nomads filled the road in their search for water and grazing ground for their camels, cattle, goats, cows, and fat-tailed sheep. Images of fat-tailed sheep have been found on temple walls dating back to Egypt's Middle Kingdom. When passing a black cow, I frequently was asked whether I wanted the jeep to stop for me to take the cow's picture. Abdellah Mohammed, who arranged the interviews with midwives and provided translation, immediately explained, "The black cow is holy. The black cow is our cow."

At one point, it occurred to me that after more than an hour on the road, we had not passed any women. Where were the women?

Abdellah explained that in traditional Afar pastoral culture, women are the keepers of the homestead, where everyday work includes taking care of the children, feeding domestic animals, carrying water over long distances, fetching firewood, and even building their "pack and go" houses that can be easily dismantled and carried on the backs of camels.

Shortly after we returned to a paved highway after being on the ancient road for more than an hour, the Megenta health care facility where TBAs work as part of the health care team popped up like a mirage. Welcomed by the facility administrator, who quickly nodded a greeting and remained seated behind a wooden desk while scribbling on a pad, I turned to Mariam Awwal Mohammed, the midwife, who signaled that our conversation could begin. Wearing a black veil that covered her face like a skirt (which her Muslim tradition requires in the presence of a man), Mariam also advocated for continuing the traditional birthing rituals and practices that elder midwives supported, which extended for 40 days after birth.

MARIAM: *The TBA always sits close to you when your days are near to seven days [before expecting to give birth] and gives care. The elder TBA who assisted me advised me to take plenty of milk and butter. If you are sick, they give*

Serra, which is the tail of [a] sheep, and they wash your body and slight[ly] massage your back.

If a mother is sick, the elder TBA stays with her until she feels well. Even if [the TBA] is called by another woman to assist, she will go to assist the other woman and then come back to you so she can give us care equally. That is rare. Usually there are some other TBAs in the locality.

She is still with the delivered women seven days later, when she will start steaming or smoking the house using different essences from leaves such as Killayto and Seganto. We have it here at the back side of the compound, and we will go and see it. The steaming is only for a mother, not for a kid, so babies will not get the smoke. A woman after delivery must stay 40 days without having any kind of sexual intercourse. She doesn't do anything, just eat and sleep, and when 40 days are finished, the midwife can help her as she washes her body in a different way with leaves. A mixture of cow or sheep dung is ground up and mixed with spices and leaves. It is put in the fire to smoke the house.

These days some women don't stay at home for 40 days. But I have never heard [of] sexual relations starting before 40 days.

Mariam paused before continuing to describe the influence of a singular midwife, Fatuma Hamadu, the "Mother" for the many women who received her integrative care. "She could not be here today because she had to leave to visit with her sick brother in the hospital," Mariam explained, as she turned to glance at Fatuma's picture, mounted in a large frame on the wall behind the administrator's desk. Mariam's descriptions of Fatuma's role in the community were similar to those described by other women I met who trusted and respected the midwives who cared for them. For example, I learned that mothers might share their deepest secrets with a midwife.

Mariam described the depth of trust and respect women had for Fatuma, whose care defines "mother of the one."

MARIAM: *There is a known Mother called Fatuma who is a highly respected mother who assists many women, and she stays with women a very long time. She brings food and clothes for those who are in need. She tells the husbands to bring good food for [their wives]. She advises women to take enough food. She never takes money. She does this care for the sake of Allah. She makes a special washing [ablution] before performing the delivery. Many babies are named by her because the community loves her. Mother Fatuma is known by the health center and works with the health center. She was taken out of this area and trained for two months. She is a member of the health committee for the health center. In our area many women want to be attended by her. She nowadays brings women to the health facility unless [an] urgent birth comes suddenly. Some women want to deliver at home because they don't want to come to the health facility for the reason that they don't want to be seen by the health professionals, especially not to be seen by men.*

I have stories to share with you about what a woman did a few days ago since we were visiting her at her home. She was telling us she will be delivered at home. Finally, when her delivery time came, she completely refused to go to the facility. Then I went to her to advise her and to take her with me to the health center. She refused. She only wanted to be delivered by Mother Fatuma. Then we called for Mother Fatuma, who assisted her at home.

After our conversation, Mariam suggested walking through a gate that opened up to the edge of the forest. There I saw a tree with a massive extended branch which Mariam talked about in ways that made it seem holy. Mariam explained that the ancient tree's leaves were a source of healing medicines and that the charcoal made from its branches was also used in ceremonies that she described. When I walked alone toward what appeared to be a place dug out for holy bathing near the tree,

Mariam suddenly became alarmed and told me to back away because I would be attacked by snakes. In a final glance at the sprawling tree that appeared to be deeply rooted in primeval sacred grounds, I could see why Mariam believed in the power of its healing leaves.

Following my last interview in Afar, I was surprised with a lunch invitation to the home of a family that I did not know. The hostess welcomed me to sit on one side of the table and instructed the male guests to sit in the seats that she assigned them on the other side of the table. I began feeling that I was a special guest of honor. At one point, the hostess washed my feet and gently placed food in my mouth by hand three times as she told me that this ritual insured that I would return. Although the ritual in Korogocho, Kenya, was different, I delighted in having a second ritual performed promising my return to the Continent.

Following lunch, when the hostess invited me to go outside with her while her daughter prepared the coffee for a coffee ceremony, the men disappeared. After several days in Afar, I learned to appreciate the coffee ceremony as a time to see the black coffeepot sitting on top of a small white stove filled with black charcoal as a symbol of Black people's strength and power. This, however, was the first time I enjoyed a coffee ceremony prepared by a woman for just women.

Once back in Addis, I had a new sense of belonging in Ethiopia that I gained from my time interviewing midwives in Wolaita Sodo and Afar. On my last morning in Ethiopia before flying to Ghana, I decided to learn more about Ethiopia and the rich spiritual practices I was just beginning to absorb. Arriving at the Ethnological Museum of the Institute of Ethiopian Studies in Addis Ababa, I was the museum's first visitor that day.

At one point, while I sat cross-legged on the museum floor reading a placard about the ancestors of the Nuer people who live in southwestern Ethiopia, I was drawn to the following:

The Nuer people who reside in southwestern Ethiopia and speak an ancient language rooted in the Nile-Saharan family celebrate Buk, a woman, as the creative force "who resides in the sky and upon the earth in rivers and streams . . . Buk's symbol is the pied crow whose brilliant black and white pilgrimage unites earth and sky." According to the Nuer story of creation, Buk's mystery is expressed in "vulnerabilities like childbirth and menstruation." Despite her vulnerabilities, "Buk participates more fully in the mysteries of life than a man."

While midwives in Afar described midwives as "mother of the one," I began to think of Buk as the "Mother of Midwives."

When I left the museum that morning to prepare for travel to Ghana, I carried with me a revelation. Just as women in Afar spoke of sharing their deepest secrets with a midwife they respected for mothering them during pregnancy, childbirth, and for weeks after, I read the placard again as I prepared to leave Addis and thought of continuing to share my secrets with Buk, whom I thought of as the First Midwife.

CHAPTER 5

Kpana

Healing Plants, Upright Birthing, Afterbirth Ceremony

Ghana is an everyday word in my vocabulary, but I never imagined that four decades after naming my daughter Ghana, a midwife would be meeting me at the airport in Kumasi, Ghana, once the capital of the Ashanti Kingdom, holding up a card with my name on it.

Seeing Ghana as their ancestral home began for many African Americans in the 1960s after Ghana became the first nation in sub-Saharan Africa to win freedom and declare independence from British colonial rule. When Kwame Nkrumah became president of the independent African nation, increasing numbers of African Americans declared Ghana as a haven for healing from the trauma of systemic racism and as a welcoming place for supporting Pan-African liberation movements and cultural work. The roll call of cultural workers and scholars who moved to Ghana in the 1960s include scholar W. E. B. Du Bois and poet Maya Angelou. While working as an illustrator for the Ghana Publishing Corporation, Tom Feelings began what became his lifetime work to document the horrors of the Middle Passage. About being in Ghana, Feelings wrote, "And I did see the joy. Africa heightened my feelings of identity. For the first time in my life, I was in the majority."

After two days of trying to make arrangements for travel to Northern Ghana, I realized that seeing Ashanti women gracefully balance their world of belongings on top of their heads gave me the confidence I needed to make a six-hour journey on the Volta Bus line to Tamale, the business capital of the Northern Region. Tikka Winner, who made the arrangements for me to meet midwives in the community of Kpana the next day, was told to look out for an African American woman wearing sneakers and carrying a large backpack.

After two busy days in Kumasi, I boarded a bus with comfortable cushioned seats and windows perfect for tourists wanting to snap photos of local markets on the six-hour ride to Tamale, the region's growing business hub. This predominantly Muslim district was once part of the Dagomba Kingdom. Established in the 11th century, at one point this empire covered more than 8,000 miles and included sections of present-day Nigeria.

At the peak of the colonial slave trade, numerous Africans were sold in Northern Ghana. That might even include my own ancestors. Today the Ghana Tourist Ministry encourages African descendants from across the diaspora who are interested in ancestral research to visit Northern Ghana. When naming my daughter Ghana, I did not know that years later DNA analysis would suggest that our ancestors came from the region that was once part of the Dagomba Kingdom.

Surrounded by traditional round huts topped with conical shaped roofs of thatch and dried straw, I met Fati Fatawu, the first midwife I interviewed in Kpana, just as the morning heat was beginning to rise. Even before our interview began, Fatawu, 39, proudly shared that she had assisted 36 women in childbirth that year and would soon be caring for the young lady standing next to her wearing an orange Lakers T-shirt neatly tucked into her brightly colored African print skirt. Speaking in Dagbani, the young pregnant mother reluctantly joined our conversation when asked why she decided to have her baby with a midwife in the village rather than go to the clinic. "I am having my baby here because I want to be near people I know," she softly explained.

Traditionally, formal greetings matter in the Kpana community, so we spent time extending greetings and paused to admire the skillful work of a young girl weaving cotton on a loom. Weaving is one of the few income-generating activities accessible to young women in the village, along with shea-butter processing and soap production. Just as the morning heat was starting to rise, Winner (who had arranged our meeting), along with myself and Jennifer Mengba, the interpreter, walked toward the primary school at the edge of the village, where we met the other midwives, Tiipang Npahiba and Fusiena Musah, who had agreed to be interviewed. All three of the village's midwives referred to themselves as traditional birth attendants, and though they made it clear that they no longer rely on practices passed on to them by their mothers and grandmothers, they refrained from discrediting "the older ways" that included using traditional medicines and birthing positions. They further explained that the government programs, however, did support the rights of families to continue honoring sacred rites surrounding the care and burial of the placenta.

Although Fatawu was familiar with traditional practices, she was emphatic about distinguishing herself as a TBA who refrains from recommending herbal medicine, and she emphasized that she adheres to the protocols mandated by the TBA training program, including requiring mothers to give birth in the dorsal position rather than using the traditional squatting or kneeling birthing traditions. (In this chapter, I refer to the women I interviewed as TBAs because that's how they chose to self-identify.) Along with recognizing the influence of TBA training on her practice, Fatawu also described how her delivery of self-care contributed to her success as a midwife.

FATAWU: *I became a TBA by myself. It happened when I was pregnant with my first child and the TBA lived in another household which was distant from my house. My delivery came so fast that it was too late to send for the TBA, so I gathered courage and delivered the baby myself. I have since delivered other women in my house and extended my service to the community. I am also able to notice the ill health of pregnant women after delivery[, for] which I take them to the Nyankpala clinic to be examined . . .*

I knew my child was almost out, and waiting for the community TBA would have harmed my baby. So I gathered the strength to deliver my child. After the delivery, I approached Apha Nurideen, the community volunteer, to talk to the health personnel so that I [could] be properly trained to offer my service.

Although Fatawu does not recommend herbal medicines such as Kagligu-tim, a medicine once frequently used by childbearing mothers in her village, she was knowledgeable about its preparation and use. Fatawu recognized that many local mothers still respected culturally based practitioners such as soothsayers and traditional healers (who are not dependent on commercial pharmaceuticals to reduce anxiety during pregnancy and birthing), and she was familiar with the location of sacred groves in the nearby forest where medicinal plants could be found. Fatawu knew practitioners who knew how to prepare black medicine—medicine which is based on botanical knowledge and experience using indigenous plants.

FATAWU: I never took any special tea during my pregnancy, but this was done during the olden days. They used to give pregnant women Kagligu-tim, a locally made black medicine which is prepared from the roots of trees. The roots are burnt into charcoal before it is ground up and mix[ed] with water to be taken by pregnant women. [In] recent time[s], nurses and health personnel have campaigned against pregnant women taking the Kagligu-tim.

They also used a leaf so people can add Tikuhum medicine to the fire to cause smoke which is believed to protect the child against evil spirits, especially children who sleep and wake up suddenly, crying a lot.

Another medicine named Nagbantogtim is a black medicine that is used to draw a circle around the baby, which becomes the baby's sleeping place till the baby grows. This medicine is believed to fight against evil spirits that may harm the child. These leaves are gotten from the trees [from] which Tikuhum and Nagbantogtim is prepared. I do not know anyone who could help locate these trees since these were old practices observed during birth.

Sometimes in cases when the woman is delayed in giving birth, they visited soothsayers to seek spiritual protection for the mother and the baby during and after delivery. These soothsayers sometimes give their preferred names to such children. Examples of these names are Yabdoo for male[s] or Yabpaga for females. In instances where no medicine is given, they only pour [a] libation with the soothsayer reciting to the gods and ancestors for protection . . .

In the traditional way, the father of the child performs [the] libation to welcome the child into the family before naming the child. This has no specific day. The child is named when the father is ready to perform the libation.

In the Muslim way, the prayer leader is invited, who slaughters a sheep and recites some prayers before naming the child. It takes seven days after delivery before the Sunnah [naming ceremony] is done. The sheep slaughtered is preferably white. The child has no name until after the seven days.

No singing or drumming is done. Food is usually prepared for the prayer leaders and the elders who attend the Sunnah naming ceremony. The prayer leader is usually their mosque prayer leader. Also, during the naming ceremony, the child's hair is shaved off. It is believed that shav-

ing off the child's hair gives him or her a new beginning of life. A special prayer is said during the slaughtering of the sheep and naming of the child.

TBAs do not have any special prayers or recite any special prayers when delivering pregnant women but only pray to God for a successful delivery of their client because it is Him [God] who has blessed them with the gift of delivery. May the delivery be successful to the glory of God's name.

Fusiena Musah, 42, who used to observe her late grandmother assisting mothers in her community, remembered the respect the village showered on her grandmother and the traditions her grandmother supported. Showing respect through words of honor, kneeling or squatting when greeting an elder, and gifting with specially prepared bars of soap, a kola nut, or a prized cut of animal meat used in the making of a traditional soup continue to be valued as gifts of appreciation far more than money by many elders. Musah explained how traditional acts of kindness and appreciation are the rewards that strengthen the bonds between the midwife and the community she serves.

Musah also described her grandmother's knowledge and use of the herbal medicine, Kagligu-tim, during pregnancy and birth. Born in Nykpala-Kukuanayi, Musah remembered learning from her grandmother, Tipaag, from an early age.

MUSAH: *Everyone respected her [Musah's grandmother]. If they saw her when walking, they followed her. They showered all kinds of blessings on her. It wasn't money. They would say words like "May you live long," and "Thank you," and "God bless you." Most people called my grandmother "Nma," followed by her name. When they prepared the meal after delivery, they would set aside special food for her.*

They would even go to her after the delivery for advice. The husbands consulted with her if the mother [was] having a problem. She [would] ask what the mother and the baby have had to eat. She [might] tell the husband to get the food or the Kagligu-tim for the mother to drink.

The Kagligu-tim was taken by women during the beginning of the seventh month of the pregnancy for strength so the baby can be strong, healthy and easy to deliver. It is also given during or after delivery for the mother to regain strength.

In the olden days, the Kagligu-tim in its powder form was mixed with water for the woman to drink. They used two empty bottles to massage the stomach from both sides. The woman [was] then asked to blow air into the bottle which aids in pushing out the placenta with pressure. However, this is no longer practiced.

Also, the Kagligu-tim is taken during pregnancy to help reduce or cure fibroids which mostly occupy space in the womb.

I could identify some of the trees used to prepare the Kagligu-tim, but not all. There were so many trees that the grandmothers used to make medicine to give to pregnant women before and after delivery when the women became weak. The Kagligu-tim is prepared from the collection of trees whose roots and leaves are obtained from the forests. The roots and leaves are brought home, where [a] libation is performed asking ancestors to purify the medicine for consumption. I can go to the forest and show you the trees. I know them when I see them, but I don't remember the names. There are older people in my community who can identify all these trees whose roots and leaves are used to prepare the Kagligu-tim.

Because of some bad outcomes, the clinic has told us to tell mothers not to take it.

Musah explained that nurses feared that the herbs some midwives recommended could lead to premature labor or other complications. In fact, the midwives were told in their training classes that it was not safe to use these medicines because they had not been deemed safe by the Western-based pharmaceutical industry, for example.

While there are ongoing studies in Ghana assessing the risks and benefits of an array of herbal medicines, the benefits of birthing in the upright birthing position have been confirmed in numerous studies. Yet midwives in Kpana explained how TBAs are instructed to only support mothers when they agree to give birth while lying flat on their backs, the preferred birthing position for a hospital delivery room table. Both Musah and Tiipang Npahiba, a midwife who is now in her 60s, remembered their grandmothers supporting mothers giving birth in the traditional upright birthing positions of kneeling or stooping.

Npahiba, the oldest of the midwives I interviewed that day, laughed when I asked her age and said that she might be in her 60s. Rather than telling time according to the Gregorian calendar, Npahiba, like other midwives I met, marked time by remembering significant events. She proudly said, "I am old enough to remember when Nkrumah became the nation's first president." When Nkrumah became president in 1957, the overwhelming majority of women in Ghana were having their babies outside of the hospital, supported by their mothers and grandmothers, who used traditional birthing positions.

NPAHIBA: *I delivered my child myself. If I called someone to come, I would have delivered the baby by the time that person got there. Late in the night, who is going to come and help you to deliver? It is not like now. People were busy with the farm. Who are you going to call to come and deliver? In those days we lived far apart. No point in calling for the TBA. By the time she comes, the baby will be there.*

I learned this from my grandmother: how to know when the baby is about to come. They used to use their bare hands—so they would take the baby with their bare hands. They know when the child is about to come. I used to follow my grandmother, who was a TBA. When my

*grandmother was doing it, I used to go with her. I walked
with my grandmother so many times. I knew I could care
for myself. I used one hand to support the buttocks and
used the other hand to catch the head.*

*I became known because I could deliver myself and the
baby would be healthy, so they called me to deliver other
ones.*

*Now we tell mothers to lie down when having their
babies, but my grandmother allowed them to squat. My
grandmother said this was an easier and faster way to
deliver.*

Both Npahiba and Musah demonstrated the kneeling and
squatting birthing positions they used when supported by their
grandmothers. "I kneeled down to deliver. That was my grandmother's preferred method of delivery because it makes it easier and faster for the baby to come out," Musah explained. She
added that the squatting position eliminated the need for exten-
sive massaging. "She only delivered pregnant women by allow-
ing them to squat," Musah said.

As I watched Musah and the other midwives authoritatively
and joyfully demonstrate the birthing positions they learned
from their grandmothers, I realized that I was watching Kpana
midwives position themselves in the birthing positions pic-
tured on ancient Egyptian temple walls and on thousands-of-
years-old birthing bricks. Recently uncovered birthing bricks
in South Abydos in Egypt's Middle Kingdom from the period
1700–1650 BC show women giving birth in an upright kneeling
birthing position using meskhnet bricks for support; the word
meskhnet is literally translated as "that which is front of birth,"
which suggests that the birthing brick is used to support the
upright birthing position.

Similar to how midwives in Kenya and Ethiopia viewed
birth, as the returning of an ancestral spirit, Musah described
a cosmological understanding of birth as an ancestral spirit
returning.

MUSAH: The grandfather goes to the soothsayer to know which of his grandfathers has come back, because they believe that any new child born is a rebirth and there are traces of its ancestor in the child. So they go to ask a soothsayer which of the grandfathers has come back. They do not mention any name to the soothsayer, but they give the characteristics of the baby. They then pour libations, and then the soothsayer throws the cowrie shells using a long stick and they ask who has returned.

In parts of Nigeria, one of the words for birthing is *ikunle,* literally translated as "kneeling." And the day of childbirth, *ojo inkunle,* is translated as the day or the birthday when an "ancestor lands on earth." In ancient Egypt, birthing was shown as part of the eternal cycle of rebirthing in illustrations on birthing bricks and wands that surrounded the mother. For example, images of Hathor, the divine Goddess of the Sky, giving birth to her son Ra, the Sun, each morning at dawn suggests that a woman becomes a goddess when giving birth.

Fatawu also explained how healers would draw a circle around the newborn, who is placed on the earth in a ritual conducted in the Kpana community to protect the baby, who they believe is suffering because of religious or magical interventions aimed at harming the newborn. This description reminded me of an ancient Egyptian illustration from the Middle Kingdom showing a similar practice.

Fatawu also described rituals regarding care for the placenta that reflect the belief that the fate of the placenta remains connected to the fate of the child. The ancient Egyptian word for placenta is translated as "the mother of humankind." The finding of a mummified placenta from thousands of years ago in a small temple has led researchers to speculate that it may have been preserved in a temple built specifically for that purpose. In the Kpana community, Fatawu explained how some families built a hut dedicated to the burial of family placentas. Her description of preparing the placenta for burial reminded me of a funerary rite.

FATAWU: The placenta is kept in a small pot called [a] Dugbila, which is made of clay. White cotton is first laid inside this pot before the placenta is placed in it. Another layer of white cotton is placed on top of the placenta before it is covered with the pot's lid. The placenta in the pot is covered well with cotton and the lid so that no particle of any form can get in touch with it. If any particle or dirt touches the placenta, it will make the child deaf or will cause hearing problems to the child. A pit is dug to the knee level to bury the placenta to keep animals away from digging it out. The child dies when dogs or pigs eat the placenta, so it should not be thrown just anywhere. The placenta is disposed of in a recognized hut built either inside or outside the house. All the children in the house have their placenta buried inside that hut.

We do not throw away dead bodies, so why do we throw away the placenta? Throwing the placenta away means the child is thrown away. This tradition is recognized in the clinics in Ghana, where the placenta is given out to the family to take home after delivery.

Before leaving, the midwives wanted to be certain that I understood the importance of the steps required in the ritual surrounding the placenta burial. As I heard the noonday call to prayer, I learned that the village prayer leader would share the steps for proper burial of the placenta. Walking back to the center of the village where elders waited, children played, and the chickens walked in and out of the smaller huts, I could see his authority in his stance even before he spoke.

Beside him, a woman stooped closed to the ground, preparing the tools needed to complete the funerary process for burial of the placenta like an attendant arranging an altar for

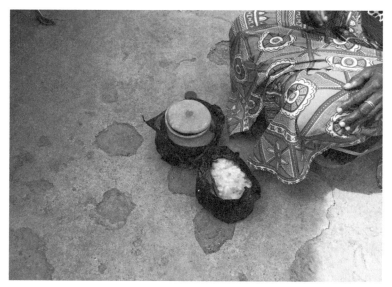

FIGURE 5.1. Kpana burial of afterbirth. A special clay pot holds the placenta. Cotton is used as a burial shroud.

the ancestors. I snapped pictures as she filled a small brown clay pot with fluffy white cotton that she pulled from a black plastic bag. The prayer leader then explained, "After the placenta is placed in the pot another layer is added."

Pointing to a small hut next to the woman preparing the pot for burial, the prayer leader continued: "We bury the pot in a hut where placentas from other family members are buried. If anything gets inside the pot, it can affect the brain and the hearing of the child. The pot is buried six feet under the ground. A man must do the job. It can't be done by a woman. If a man is not around, a young boy close by can be asked to do the job" (see figure 5.1).

As I listened and watched the funerary process for burial of the placenta, I bowed my head in prayer. Like griots known for the drumming of the ancestral history of the Dagomba Empire, the midwives I met in the Kpana community raised up the spirits of midwives in their midwifery lineage like chroniclers of history. That's when I understood that I was standing on venerated ground where the placentas—"the mothers of humankind" as described by ancient Egyptians—that fed my ancestors and others of African descent who were forcefully separated from their homeland were buried. I was standing on ground enriched with abundant "mother of humankind" spirit.

CHAPTER 6

Ejura

Lineage Apprenticeships, Spiritual Cleansings, Born with the Gift

When I returned to Kumasi, Ghana—the capital of the Asante Region—the explosion of pride and rejoicing in the celebrations of the 20th anniversary of the enstoolment of King Asantehene Otumfuo Osei Tutu II was palpable in the drumming and dancing I witnessed. Although the king's role is now ceremonial, the powerful cultural traditions within the Asante Region live on not only in celebration of the "Golden Stool," said to house the spirit of the Asante people, but also in the keeping of traditions and rituals. Dating back as far as oral and written records show, these traditions and rituals recognize a Supreme Being and honor a host of deities, the ancestors, and the forces of nature.

While I was in Kumasi, my host Gertrude Annan Aidoo, who heads the nurse midwife program at the Komfo Anokye Hospital, made her office a space for my immersion into Asante culture—she taught me about hair braiding, selected traditional kente cloth to make into a suit I could wear back at home when talking about my work in Ghana, and taught me about the many uses of cocoa leaves hanging from the trees that I could easily reach from the balcony outside her office.

Over a welcoming lunch of chicken, fufu, and what Black folks in the US call black-eyed peas, one of the nurse midwives asked about the purpose of my visit. "I will be interviewing midwives in Accra," I said, expecting a nod of approval. To my surprise, she said, "They are all dead," referring to the traditional midwives.

I knew that the sprawling hospital, the second largest in Ghana—named for Komfo Anokye, who was born in 1955 and is credited with establishing the Asante Kingdom—is the Ashanti Region's major provider of maternity care for mothers and babies. I also knew that Kwame Nkrumah had dismantled the segregated colonial hospital system of Ghana where Africans had cared for Africans and Europeans had cared for Europeans. Now, on the hospital grounds, countless families of all backgrounds waited overnight, resting on mats under large hospital-installed electric fans, and waiting for news about their newborns..

"Don't worry," Gertrude quickly interjected. "We will find midwives for you to interview."

Two days later, I was headed to Ejura in the northern Ashanti Region. That meant squeezing into the backseat of a packed van next to a breastfeeding mother who carried with her, in a small cardboard box, a live chicken that nibbled on my toes throughout the trip. Somehow, I stayed centered and channeled my energy to completely still all body movements so I wouldn't disturb the baby.

I met Matilda Ibrahim and Hoya Baformene three hours later in a town where the major attraction was the local hospital. Estra Hopeson, a young graduate of the Kumasi Hospital nursing program who works at the Ejura hospital, hosted the interviews in her home, where I was also invited to spend the night. The two midwives I met in Ejura confirmed that local training programs are dismantling many traditional midwifery practices, as they are unwilling to support integrative birthing-care models that recognize the value of social supports, mental and emotional balancing through spiritual connections, and a range of healing practices that respect interconnections between body, mind, and spirit. The midwives described the use of traditional herbs that they previously included in their practices. While adapting to new requirements, Ejura midwives have not lost respect for themselves.

In Ejura, the hospital is demanding that midwives bring all mothers to the hospital to have their babies. Both of the Ejura midwives I spoke with began their midwifery practices in their home villages. Even after moving to Ejura, Ibrahim did not identify herself as a midwife until her community's TBA died and community members asked her to take over her practice. Later, Ibrahim said that a local assemblyman recommended that she go to the hospital and take a three-day training course offered to TBAs.

Like other midwives in Ghana, Ibrahim (see figure 6.1) tells time in terms of before and after independence. As a way to gauge her age, Ibrahim said she remembered President Nkrumah's signature 1961 Akosombo Dam project, which supplied a large area with electrical power for the first time. Proudly announcing that she was the mother of 12 children, she added that her first three children had been born before Ghana became an independent nation, so I estimated her birth year around 1949, the same year I was born.

Born in Krache Dente, home of the Krache Dente Shrine in the eastern part of Ghana, Ibrahim grew up in a region that is home to one of the oldest religious institutions of ancestral worship on the Continent. Now a tourist destination, the Krache Dente Shrine once drew Asante's chiefs and other traditional military leaders from long distances to consult with Krache Dente's powerful oracle.

Ibrahim was the only midwife I interviewed whose initiation into the practice of midwifery was not guided by a woman; her practice began under her father's tutelage. She described how her father, as a widely known spiritual healer and ritual specialist, would use the throwing of cowrie shells as part of a spiritually guided process to determine whether an illness was psychological or physical. Ibrahim also explained how her father prescribed medicines based on spiritual guidance and interpretation of rituals.

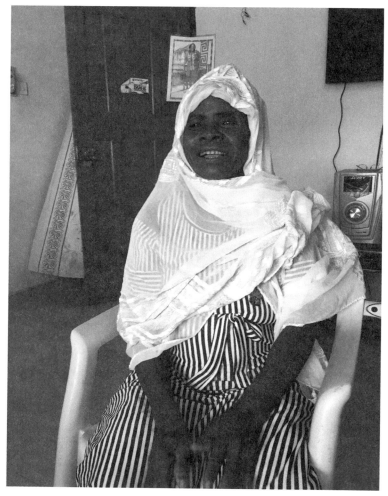

FIGURE 6.1. Matilda Ibrahim in the home of Estra Hopeson

IBRAHIM: *My father was a ritualist who assisted women who wanted children, and he also gave medicine to women to assist them in having a smooth delivery. If any woman had complications during delivery, my father was called upon to assist. So I picked this work up from my father.*

After my father applied the drugs on the mother's abdomen to help her delivery, he would leave, and I would have to assist the woman with delivery. I started being a mid-wife because of my father . . .

He wasn't directly involved in assisting with the deliveries. My father was the only man in our village who attended to pregnant women, and he gave medicines during pregnancy and through to delivery.

Years later, after moving to Ejura, Ibrahim became a midwife. She respected the elder midwife in practice before beginning practice in her new community. Ibrahim explained how midwifery practices are passed through the family line.

IBRAHIM: *There were other women in my community who were TBAs. It is handed down the family line so when one dies, the work is handed down to the daughter to take it up. One of my sisters is currently a TBA—but at the time my father was teaching me, all my siblings were younger. I am the oldest, so I was the only one old enough at that time.*

When I first came into this community [Ejura], I wasn't practicing as a TBA until the TBA in the community died and I was asked to take her place, so I did . . .

Similar to other midwives I interviewed, Ibrahim believes her ability to support herself without assistance through labor and birth was the first step to becoming a midwife. In a culture where psychological and emotional stresses are believed to have the power to negatively affect birthing outcomes, Ibrahim added that caring for herself during labor and birth protected her and her newborn from being harmed by members of her polygamous community at a time when she was most vulnerable.

IBRAHIM: *I give birth on my own without assistance. I gave birth to all my 12 children on my own. Whenever I am in labor, nobody gets to know. I go about my normal duties and before my rivals [other wives] in the house would know . . .*

I never had any problems when I was having my babies. When you are pregnant you need to eat a lot of greens, and whenever you have an appetite for other food and fruits you can eat it. Sometimes my father told me not to eat certain foods, but I still ate them. But most importantly I ate a lot of vegetables, so they said that is why I was able to give birth easily.

Some people under normal circumstances experience some difficulties during labor but I have never experienced that; neither did my mother.

We both give birth to our children easily and on our own . . . We buy our razor blade so after delivery, we cut the umbilical cords before we call our husband or someone to help bathe the baby. This is the case for me and my mother . . .

It is my aunty who could've assisted me in delivery, but before she gets to the place, I have already given birth and the placenta is already out.

I squat during my deliveries. On my last delivery I was lying on my back. My mother buried the placenta. The other women in the community cannot deliver on their own, so they are assisted by the TBAs.

Born in Koro in the northern Asante Region, Madam Hoya Baformene also discussed how she successfully gave birth without additional support and why she preferred the squatting position. Estimating her age to be in the 60s, Baformene said about her heritage and ethnic group, "We are Sisala." She added that after birth the newborn infant "is presented to the gods and the eldest man in the house pours libations and gives the name."

BAFORMENE: *When I am delivering on my own, I sit in a chair, and when the baby is about coming out, I squat, but when someone assists me during delivery I squat down. I don't lie down during my deliveries.*

If I lay down during delivery, especially if I am delivering on my own, how can I catch the baby when it is coming out? That is why I sit on a chair.

Because we don't deliver at the hospital, we prefer squatting so that if the position of the baby is not right, we can push it into the right position to reduce tears.

When I am delivering [a] baby, the mothers also squat. The one in labor holds my shoulders and another person holds the mother's waist while she pushes so when the baby comes out I squat and catch it.

When you touch and examine the abdomen you will know if it is time for her to push. If the baby is not positioned well, you can also know and position it well before telling her to push.

I will know. When I touch the stomach and the baby is ready to come out, I will know, then I let her squat and push.

Baformene never received formal training as a TBA and credits her mother for the valuable lessons that prompted her to become a midwife.

BAFORMENE: *My mother was born with the gift of assisting deliveries, so nobody taught her. You know in the olden days, it was common for people to be born with such gifts, so she taught me how to do it.*

I learned a lot from my mother before I got married. She taught me how to assist someone during delivery. I couldn't follow my mother for a long period because when she finished teaching me I got married, and I started giving birth.

The main thing I learned from my mother was that all her children had died except for four of us and we were all girls; all her male children had died. She had given birth to 12 children and four of us were left, and now there are only two of us left.

So when she told me about the death of my sisters and brothers, I kept it in mind and used it.

As I learned in Kumasi, the practices of traditional midwives are rapidly being phased out across the Asante Region. Baformene has not attended any births as a midwife for more than four years. Nevertheless, she continued to vow for the efficacy of the herbal medicines she'd previously used.

BAFORMENE: *When the blood is flowing, I used a special herb. As I sit here, you will not be able to name the herb I am talking about even if I showed you. Just know, I apply the herbs on her abdomen and the bleeding stops. I don't know the Twi [Akan] name for the herb. I only know the name of the herb in my local language, and you would not know it if I mention the name. It is called Soolo. I apply it by massaging the pregnant woman's stomach with it.*

Even though she no longer continues her practice as a midwife, Baformene remained proud of her herbal knowledge and offered to provide samples of the plants that she described like the midwives in Kenya and Northern Ghana.

BAFORMENE: *The herb we gave to them in pregnancy is from the root of a tree. We uproot the roots of the tree, wash it well, and grind it for them to drink. It gives them strength during pregnancy and delivery.*

But during delivery you would have to give a very small quantity with enough water, and then she would deliver easily. I don't know its name in the Twi [Akan] language. In my local language it is called Banmorna.

It really works very well. If you had told me earlier, I would've brought some for you.

Baformene also provided examples of how midwives were rewarded in the past. "It was only the soap that they gave me. They are supposed to give me soap, kola nuts, and herbs." The former midwife continued, "I used the herb to wash my face." In Ghana, kola nuts are gifted as symbols of peace, unity, and love, and are also viewed as symbols that mark the beginning of life.

Still practicing as a midwife, Ibrahim agreed that midwives in the past and now continue to be respected and gifted by women for the care they provide and that the herbal medicines she used in the past do work. Ibrahim, however, adamantly denied using any herbal medicines now. "What I am explaining is that because of modern medicine, I have stopped giving them because people will complain that I have been giving herbal drugs," she said. "I wouldn't be able to talk much about them to you now because I have stopped using them so I can't remember them." Still respectful of her father's wisdom and practices, Ibrahim described how her father prepared an herbal mixture that he used in a ritual of purification that he prepared for her after completing the work of assisting a birthing mother.

IBRAHIM: *When someone came to my father, he consulted the gods by throwing cowrie shells to determine whether the problem was spiritual or medical before he decided on what to do for the person. There were no doctors at the time, so he used the herbs. If the problem was spiritual, he would give the mother some concoction to drink and also give her some herbs to put into fire, so that the smoke [would] drive the bad spirit away. We have lost all those herbs because of modern medicine. I don't know the name of the herb, but it used to be in the north, and it is added to the bark of another tree from the north to prepare that herb for burning.*

I don't use the herbal drugs. The doctors and nurses say it is bad, but I think it was a good thing that the doctors and nurses could've learned from. From the olden days, it is the herbal drugs that we have been using, so there is nothing wrong with it. One of the nurses at the hospital was even telling me [that] her mother is a TBA and sometimes uses herbs, so there is nothing wrong with the herbal drugs. If someone wants to conceive or is in labor and having difficulty in delivering, my father knew how to give her an herbal drug to assist her to conceive or deliver . . .

Currently in Ghana, the Mampong Centre for Plant Research, which is affiliated with the University of Ghana at Legon, has gained international recognition for research and development of herbal products from study of locally grown plants. During the years of Kwame Nkrumah's presidency, Oku Ampofo, a medical doctor and renowned artist, planted the seeds for ongoing research that taps into the wisdom of timeless healers and traditional practitioners, including midwives. Prior to leaving Ghana, I visited the Mampong Centre, where there is continuing interest in the study of plant-based medicine used by traditional midwives. The Ejura midwives expressed interest in contributing to the development of a project that includes the study of plants used by Ibrahim's father and Baformene in the past. "People would come from miles away," Baformene explained, "seeking advice from my father."

Ibrahim also described how her father used rituals and spiritual cleansings to restore balance after a midwife completes her work of assisting a mother and baby. As she explained, her father used a chicken in a cleansing ritual because animal blood is believed to have spiritual powers.

IBRAHIM: *My father performed spiritual cleansings for us—the TBAs—because we need to be spiritually strong for this work we do. So he takes a fowl for us so that he can wash our faces spiritually so that we don't get blind as a result of this work we do. So after every delivery he gives me a concoction to wash my face with. After every delivery, I take a fowl—I put the fowl down and wash my*

*face with the concoction in front of the fowl for special
cleansing to prevent me from going blind. After this, I rear
the fowl.*

As I listened, I thought about how contemporary practitioners rigorously sanitize themselves in order to be protected from contamination during delivery through vigorous cleansing and the wearing of gloves, mask, and gowns. But there are no rituals for restoration and spiritual healing after the strenuous procedures, exhaustive work, or health threats that health care providers face during a pandemic.

Although the practices of traditional midwives are rapidly declining, Ibrahim remains an active midwife in her community. Estimating that she sometimes delivers as many as 20 babies in a busy month, Ibrahim said that they seek her services because they know "I am friendly and approachable. That is why they prefer coming to me." She added, "I like laughing, so they like coming to me." Ibrahim, who was once Catholic and is now a follower of the Islamic faith, added, "I do what I do because if the person is in difficulty and asks for my assistance, how can I say I wouldn't help?"

Baformene, however, is unable to continue her practice, as she sadly explained.

BAFORMENE: *Now I have been asked to stop delivering
mothers at home. That is why I bring them to the facility. I
stopped four years ago. When they put up the health center
at Homako and brought [in] a trained nurse midwife, she
asked me to stop delivering. My children also didn't support what I was doing, so when the midwife asked me to
stop, I stopped.*

*All I have to say is that I really wish I could be working as a TBA again, because if I were a TBA my daughter's
issue wouldn't have happened. I would've known how to
help my daughter during her labor so that she wouldn't
have lost her baby.*

Tears welled up in her eyes as she said, softly, "It really disturbs me. I could have saved the baby."

Although her daughters have urged her to give up her midwife practice, she wants to continue being a midwife.

> BAFORMENE: *I wish doctors would train me and allow me to practice as a TBA because currently I have two daughters who are pregnant, and I can help them during their delivery. When they are due and the baby is not positioned well, I can reposition the baby to make for an easy delivery. I really wish I would be allowed to practice as a TBA. Personally, if I were allowed to be a TBA again, I would do it.*

Having already said farewell to Ibrahim, I prepared to end my conversation with the last midwife I would interview during my five weeks on the Continent. Unexpectedly, Baformene invited me to walk with her through the village back to the road. Hopeson, the interpreter, explained that by my walking with her, the community would see that I was honoring her.

Baformene also promised to bring samples of the herbs that she used to give mothers so that I could take them to the Mampong Centre, to test them for their efficacy. Also unexpected was her promise of a gift of a sample of the charcoal that she now makes as a business. The Sisala are famous for the making of charcoal. Unfortunately, another meeting could not be arranged, because I was leaving early the next morning to catch the van back to Kumasi, as I would soon be leaving Ghana.

Returning to Kumasi the next morning, I was once again in the midst of Asante celebrations. As I prepared for my departure to Accra to fly back to the States, Gertrude Annan Aidoo, the nurse midwife who was my host and navigator in helping to arrange interviews in Ghana, surprised me as she carried out her own impromptu naming ceremony after learning that I was born on a Saturday. She spoke like an honorary elder when she said, "Your day name is Ama." Although no libations were poured, we danced. Gertrude taught me the basic steps of the antelope, the adowa, a dance traditionally performed by women at funerals, festivals, and other ceremonial events.

While in Accra, Ghana, I met E. Ofori Akyea, an academic and historian who described elaborate naming ceremonies among the Ewe people (a Gbe ethnic group, the largest population of which is in Ghana) who live along the Atlantic Coast. According to Ewe traditions, before an infant is carried outdoors on the seventh day, the mother's house is swept, the birth fire ashes removed, and a new fire lit. Then, water is thrown onto the thatch roof of the mother's hut so that water can drip down from the eves of the roof onto the mother and baby as a ceremonial blessing. Ofori continued by explaining that "the person carrying out the ceremony dips his finger into a glass of water and then dips his finger into a glass containing alcohol. After placing a drop of each of the liquids into the baby's mouth, the ritual specialist then says to the baby, "Let its words be true. If you took alcohol, say so." On the Continent, birth traditions are a Pan-African cultural institution that ranks with initiation, marriage, and burial rituals. Although many of these traditions did not survive the transatlantic slave trade, I remembered how midwives I met in Alabama succeeded in adapting and continuing aspects of naming ceremonies similar to those that midwives and Akyea described.

Before leaving Accra to return to New York, I also visited the W. E. B. Du Bois Museum, the former house where Du Bois and his wife lived as he, then in his 90s, continued work on the Africana encyclopedia. When leaving the museum grounds, I was drawn to a lawn sale in the museum yard. My only purchase that afternoon was a pair of cotton pants that exploded in brilliant green and orange leaves. Whenever I wore the pants in Accra, at least one person would stop to tell me that the print on the pants is called "good beads don't rattle," Ahwenepa, referring to the fact that nothing needs to be said to see the beauty and strength found in the pattern. The midwives I met in Ejura have the inner beauty and strength of good beads, and so did the midwives I interviewed decades earlier in Alabama.

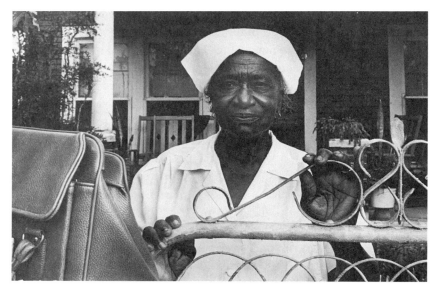

FIGURE 7.1. Aunt Shugg Lampley in uniform, peeking over a gate in New Brockton, Alabama. Image permission by © Chester Higgins. Courtesy of the Bruce Silverstein Gallery.

CHAPTER 7

Montgomery

Massage, Birthing Prayers, Burial of the Placenta

Decades before interviewing traditional midwives in Africa, I spent six months in Alabama listening to the stories of a last generation of Black lay midwives who preserved and continued culturally rich birthing traditions. In 1981 I never imagined that 40 years later I would travel to Kenya, Ghana, and Ethiopia to document parallels between birthing traditions on the Continent and the practices that had been passed on to Alabama midwives by their elders and ancestors, some of whom had been born in Africa. My conversations with midwives in Africa confirmed that despite the horrors of the Middle Passage, the era of enslavement, Jim Crow segregation, eugenics, and unrelenting biases against Black women, the Alabama midwives I had met had succeeded in preserving a way of birthing that had its roots in the Continent, continued to be spiritually based and holistic, and saved lives.

In 1976 the Alabama State Health Department stopped issuing new lay-midwife permits or renewing existing ones, part of a campaign that succeeded in eliminating an institution that once included white and Indigenous midwives as well.

Of the more than 150 midwives licensed to practice as midwives that year, all identified as Black except for one. Using the first statewide listing of lay midwives compiled by Alabama's health department, I contacted 50 lay midwives who agreed to be interviewed. In Montgomery, I also interviewed a prominent minister and civil rights activist, George Washington Carver Richardson, who remembered his grandmother's midwife practices in Gordo, Pickens County, Alabama.

While African culture was sustained in the US through music, dance, architecture, foodways, and burial practices, less has been written about retentions of the African traditions surrounding pregnancy and birth. Fortunately, midwives in Alabama lived to tell the story of how midwives of African descent reflected the wisdom, fortitude, genius, innovation, determination, and spirituality of their ancestors and community elders who passed on to them timeless birthing traditions. On the Continent and in Alabama, many midwives solidified their birthing practices in their religious beliefs. Because there were no boundaries in their ways of caring, some midwives not only provided support and guidance at the time of birth but also became a source of lifetime support, inspiration, and hope in their community.

Plans for my 1981 trip to Alabama made the CBS 6 o'clock news. At the car showroom, as I decided to purchase a stickshift Honda Civic as ideal for navigating the back roads of the Black Belt, I noticed TV cameras as a reporter focused on the uptick in Americans buying foreign-made cars. When the CBS reporter asked why I was trading in my Dodge Dart for a Honda Civic, I explained that I was going to interview Black midwives in Alabama, a state that in the 1980s promoted itself as the "cradle of the Confederacy." The interview ended with my saying that I would be traveling on back roads with Jersey license plates in a state where Blacks were murdered because they tried to register to vote; I needed a reliable car.

Deciding to live in Montgomery, I rented a small furnished house with a yard that even had a clothesline wire pinned between two poles, which provided color to the yard when I hung out clothes to dry. My first week there, my neighbor showed off her southern hospitality when she began dropping by on Fridays with fresh-caught fish, cleaned and ready to fry. A few blocks away, Lily Baptist Church offered the perfect Sunday-morning mix of Black gospel and spirituals for finding the peace of mind I had found in breathing exercises and meditations in yoga classes before moving to Alabama. I later learned how midwives on the Continent described chants, invocations, intuition, and religiously based traditional healers as among the ways that spirituality infused their practices. But years before going to Africa, I learned how deeply interwoven prayer and other expressions of faith are among nearly all the Black midwives I interviewed in Alabama. Grandmothers and great-grandmothers born in the era of enslavement contributed to how significantly spiritual practices shaped the institution of southern Black midwifery practice.

I met Mary Taylor, 70, the first midwife I interviewed in Montgomery, in her home, not long after arriving there. A longtime Montgomery resident, Taylor introduced me to Elvira Johnson and Vera Poole, who had also practiced as midwives in Montgomery County for decades. The three agreed that midwifery was not a vocation that they had chosen, but that they were initiated into the practice of midwifery by a singular midwife who was a mother, grandmother, or an extended family member. The midwife Taylor trained with was also the midwife who attended her in childbirth.

> TAYLOR: *I had all my children before I started being a midwife. I have three. The oldest one was born in 1928. And the second in 1930. And the third in 1932. Oh yeah, I had a midwife, nothing but a midwife. The same one, and she's living now. Her name is Liza Weaver. I think her age is 110. First midwife I had and is still living. She's the one that knew I'd be a midwife. She wanted me to be a midwife because she was getting old and she wanted to learn me. And that's how I started working with her.*
>
> *When I started being a midwife at that time, they did not have clinics. And all the babies—most of the babies*

delivered then—was by a midwife. All the cases that she would have, she would carry me with her because I did all her writing. She couldn't read and write. I can't tell how many years I went out with her until she just got tired and stopped. She was the midwife. And she started her work when she had her own babies because they were born and she didn't have nobody. And so she cut the cord herself with a knife; she was the first one that she ever waited on.

"Waiting on mothers" was one of the terms midwives in Alabama used to describe their work. Seeing their roles as serving and caring for woman, the phrase *waiting on women* aptly described how they viewed their traditional noninterventional roles in the birthing process; their hands were their primary tools. They learned how to use their hands effectively and skillfully through apprenticeships.

While sitting on Taylor's front porch, Poole told me she retired from her lay-midwifery practice in 1962, but she clearly remembered how a family elder, her mother-in-law, chose her to enter the practice. Even though she initially resisted becoming a midwife, she finally decided to follow elders to learn the midwife practice. Poole laughed as she recalled the conversation with her grandmother: "I told her I was too young to look up under a mother's coat, but she kept saying 'Daughter, I'm going down. I want you to take my place.'" The tradition Poole described of being chosen to follow a senior midwife in the community is a long-standing practice in communities across the diaspora as well.

Unlike doctors, who often see their roles as managing or coordinating care, midwives I met in Montgomery and in other parts of Alabama described their roles as providing a service to women that emanated from a spiritual call to midwifery practice that might come to them through a dream or vision. For midwives, similar to traditional midwives on the Continent, religious beliefs and spirituality influenced every aspect of their lives, including "waiting on women." For midwives in Alabama, the Spirit they called on was Jesus. One Alabama midwife described becoming a midwife like a religious testimony. Midwives sometimes described their decision to "wait on mothers" as a spiritual calling. Once receiving the "call," they began an apprenticeship with a senior midwife.

> POOLE: *So every time she'd go see about a patient, I'd go. If the baby comes or not comes, I'd go with her for about two years. And, she told me that there is another midwife around here named Lizzie Weaver. And said, "When you get ready to go out, you call Miss Weaver and let her go with you." Well, I did. I carried Miss Weaver with me, and Miss Weaver showed me and told me what to do. And I've been going on by myself ever since.*

Midwives who apprenticed with senior midwives also heard stories from elders in their families about the use of herbal medicines to promote overall well-being. Vera Johnson, a former midwife and now an octogenarian, remembered how her family relied on her uncle as a plant doctor. For example, he became widely known for making medicines from yellow-top weeds that he picked from the side of the road to make a tea used to treat malaria.

> JOHNSON: *And my uncle, he was really an herb doctor. He could go out in the woods and get some herbs and make medicines. We were talking a few weeks ago about the different teas he used to bring us. Didn't know what a doctor was. No. But the biggest thing they had was malaria fever back in them days, and chills and fever, and they knew how to go out there in the road and get them old yellow weeds and boil them and bathe you in them and give you a spoonful to drink, and that'd knock it out . . .*
> *My great-grandmother was a slave, but then my mother and them wasn't, and my grandmothers on both sides, they were slaves. They would talk about it and tell us how they*

> had to serve the Lord by praying over a pot of water to catch the sound . . . But they knew there was a God, and they would have their meeting. They sang and prayed . . .
>   They had herbs, and they had doctors too in that time. But wasn't many doctors. And I remember hearing Grandmama saying when the slaves had a baby, they just send someone out to the field to cut the baby's cord and tie it with some black thread. And the baby, when he got old enough, she come on back to the field.

Recalling her own birthing experience, Johnson remembered the influence of Weaver, who cared for her during labor and birth. Weaver supported her giving birth in the upright position, which was similar to how midwives I met on the Continent described how they supported the upright birthing position.

> JOHNSON: Well, she'd [Weaver] have me put on some water to wash her hands in a kettle. I was living with my mother, and she knew how to have a kettle of water, an old black kettle, sitting there in front of the fire and the wash pan. And they had old quilts and things at the time for you to deliver on, but now you've got to have paper, sterile pads, and things for them to deliver on. I delivered—the first one I delivered was on my knees, and the next one I delivered was on the bed.

Years later as a midwife, Johnson also supported the mother's birthing-position choice whenever possible rather than restricting them to the dorsal position, which health department training courses often mandated. Mothers giving birth witnessed family members or neighbors who had used the upright birthing position during birth and wanted to emulate the position that they knew worked for them. Some of the midwives I interviewed explained how they would not want to give birth lying flat on their back because it made birthing harder.

JOHNSON: I'd let them [mothers] walk around or lay down. If they were sleepy, I let them lay down and go to sleep until just about time. I could tell when the pains were getting closer and closer. Then I'd let them get up and walk around then. Then some of them would want to get on the floor and some wanted to stay in the bed. I let them do like they wanted to do 'cause they are the ones that had to have the baby. If they wanted to get on their knees, it's all right. If they wanted to lay on the floor, it was all right; and if they wanted to get in the bed, it was all right.

While Johnson learned from both Weaver and her own birthing experience skills and practices that worked to promote the best possible outcomes, she described how she tapped into her own deeply ingrained spiritual practices to help keep her focus in providing care for the mother during labor and birth. The earliest stages of labor until the cervix is fully dilated—which is when a mother begins pushing out her baby—can last six to eight hours or even longer. Midwives I met on the Continent described how women gathered outside the hut where a mother would give birth to collectively chant and pray; midwives I met with in Alabama described how they lifted up their own voices in prayer.

JOHNSON: Oh yeah, I have prayed many prayers for them to deliver and for them to be calm and easy. And you know, God would calm them down. And they'd have such a nice, normal birth. And I prayed hardest for them when it's their first baby, but them that done had children, they already knew the way and knew what to expect.

While some midwives on the Continent described communicating with the ancestors in rituals surrounding birth, midwives in Alabama talked mostly about Jesus praise songs. The spirituals, songs, hums, and moans, however, that I heard in the churches I visited in my time in Alabama preserve some of

the cadences and rhythms of the music of their African ancestors. Despite separation from their ancestral Continent, there
were infants born in enslavement who surely heard in a lullaby
a song hummed by an ancestor still in the homeland. Mary Taylor explained how the prayers she carries with her to the birthing space are not locked into a specific religious faith.

Another midwife, Carrie Morris, explained how spirituality led her to become a midwife and how Christian prayer and
revelations not only guided her midwifery practice but were
a powerful force in every aspect of her everyday life. Morris
explained that she briefly apprenticed with Kate, an experienced midwife. In Alabama, I met midwives who had attended
thousands of births as well as midwives who only occasionally
assisted mothers with birthing. What connected their practices
was their belief that God deserved the credit for their success
as midwives.

> MORRIS: *Well, the business, it come to me overnight, but it
> had dwelled with me about a month. Every time I would to
> go to sleep or something, I could see myself helping some-
> body. It just kept talking to me. Telling me, "You go ahead
> and you can do it." So I called and I asked Kate [a commu-
> nity midwife Morris knew] could I go around with her . . .
> She said, "You want to become a midwife?" I said, "Yes, I
> do." She said, "Well, all right, I'll learn you." So I went out
> with Kate for about a month. I went out with her about
> five times. Then she said, "Well, now you can go on your
> own." So, I said, "Thank you." And I turned around and
> thanked God 'cause if it hadn't been for Him, I wouldn't
> have never been one. There's nothing I do—I don't go into
> nothing unless Jesus Christ goes with me, not a thing. I
> don't open my car door unlessen I ask the Lord, please give
> me strength to open my door and go with me. I sure do.
> That's the way I work—with me and the Lord. You just
> have to trust in God. I do because I haven't run into no*

dangers, not yet, and I thank God for it. I ain't never run into no danger, not yet.

For Taylor as well, the protocol for entering the birthing space required grounding herself in prayer first.

TAYLOR: *When someone calls me and tells me to come and wait on them, I get on my knees and pray. It's a prayer to the Lord to able them to deliver. Most of them, I'd always tell them when they notify me, when they first start getting into labor, "Get your mother. If you can't get your mother, get one of your friends because it's not good to be alone by yourself."*

And then the whole time I'm working with them, I talk to my master. Then when the baby be born, everything is all right. I be talking, you know, praise. Be praising God. I talk sometimes, not out loud, so not to disturb the mother. But sometimes I may say "Thank you, Jesus. Thank you, Jesus." I'll be saying that so the mother will start saying it. Get them to say, "Thank you, Jesus." Because that's something I love to do. Praise God. I go to all churches, not just my own. I go to the Baptist, Church of Christ, Seventh-day Adventist, Methodist, anywhere they're serving the Lord. If I don't have a meeting at my church, I'll go.

Empowered by her faith, Taylor described how prayer helped her remain focused when faced with complications, such as delivering twins and having to soften the cervix to prevent tears or to release the center piece, "the placenta." Taylor explained, "Keep massaging it 'til you can get it loose. You massage them on the side. That's how them old midwives learned me how to massage it."

Being skillful in ways to position the baby for optimal birthing was described by Johnson as "rubbing the mother." Johnson said, "I have never tried to turn the baby. Uh uh, no. Because if

I thought the baby was crossways, I'd keep on rubbing them 'til finally he wakes up and turns his self."

Unexpectedly, George Washington Carver Richardson, longtime pastor of Hutchinson Missionary Baptist Church in Montgomery, provided a detailed description of how his grandmother incorporated massage into her practice as a midwife in Gordo, Pickens County, Alabama. Richardson said he was raised by his grandmother and even breastfed by her. Her hopes were that he would become a doctor. Known for referring to the hands of his grandmother in his Sunday-morning prayers and sermons as holding spiritual power, Richardson, like other Black ministers I met, honored and respected midwives.

Gwenn Patton, lifetime Montgomery resident and activist who headed the Student Nonviolent Coordinating Committee (SNCC) Women's Liberation Committee at the peak of the 1960s civil rights movement, suggested that I interview Richardson because she had heard many of his moving testimonies to his grandmother, whom he describes as a mother to him. Also a civil rights activist, Richardson had worked closely with Martin Luther King in helping to organize the Selma to Montgomery march in 1963 and later survived a brutal physical attack by the Ku Klux Klan, when he was left on the road to die; Richardson survived the attack by a white supremacist terrorist group and was the first Black person to run for mayor in Bessemer, Alabama.

When Richardson spoke about his grandmother's healing hands, his eyes appeared to gaze through spiritual waters and roll back decades of time. As a nine-year-old, when accompanying his grandmother, Richardson assisted her in small ways, such as wiping a mother's forehead as labor pains intensified when his grandmother began massaging the parturient mother.

In this passage, Richardson's rhythmic mm-hmms and uh-huns are included because they provide the kind of poetic punctuations found in the delivery of many of the sermons I heard when visiting Black churches with midwives in Alabama.

RICHARDSON: *Twice I went out with her to assist her,
because at one time she was just ill and she could not
really handle a lot of things, so she asked me to go with
her. My grandmother, because I was her oldest grandson
and mostly her favorite, she kind of pulled me along on a
lot of things. She wanted me to be a doctor. She had a lot
of dreams about that. She just took me along. But I really
never thought about going into it, per se, other than just
assisting her, mm-hmm . . .*
    *I guess that [massage] was kind of the trademark at
that time. I did not know really what was going on until
later on, until my mother got into the business, but she
would oftentimes massage her [the mother's] stomach and
move her stomach around and things like that. You know,
her thighs, to keep her from having cramps. This kind of
thing. Mm-hm. Even back then, olive oil had kind of a
religious tone to it. It was used many times in religion to
really, you know, to anoint and for prayer and meditation.
My grandmother, many times when she—before she used
oil—would pray, and then she would use that particular
oil. Before she massaged the mother, she would pray and
read scriptures constantly while the mother's in pain. So I
can't help but think that there was some religious significance to it, mm-hmm.*

In the deep tones of a minister's voice slowly rising in vol-
ume and intensity and finally reaching a crescendo, Richardson
explained how his grandmother managed a complicated birthing case by employing her sensitive hand skills and technical
and spiritual strength.

RICHARDSON: *Well, she had twins one time to deliver, and
seems as if she couldn't get them turned properly. And she
worked very hard with the mother. And she oftentimes
talked about this like it was her big moment. I don't know*

what she did, but I know that it worked her very hard because she kept every so often, according to time—she would time herself—and she would go there and work with the stomach of the mother with her hands and kept just bathing her down. And whereas other times she wouldn't do it with a system or with some kind of consistency, now she had some consistency in doing it. And every hour on the hour or minute or however she chose to do it, she would just work with that mother and work with that mother and work with that mother and work with that mother. And she had to push one baby around and get the other one to come first—she oftentimes talked about that. And then when they finally came, both of them came breeched. And that was real difficult because then—she had a problem of trying to keep the baby's neck from being broken. And she thought probably the second baby would come normal, but it came breeched, and she had to reshape the second baby's head after it had gotten here.

Her hands became beautiful when she was doing the work on the mother. She had circular motions, and her hands—her hands looking like the hands of God.

Living in rural Pickens County, Richardson's grandmother continued to incorporate the ritual of burying the placenta following birth, a ceremony she may have learned from her ancestors; research shows that this practice existed on the Continent, as I came to know from nurse midwives in the US who had previously worked on the Continent. In 1981 I learned that new health department rules led some midwives to keep hidden their support of timeless rituals to bury the afterbirth, particularly in urban communities. Richardson at the time spoke with the same kind of reverence for proper burial of the placenta as the Muslim minister I met decades later in the Kpana community, who described the importance of adhering to local traditions regarding burial of the afterbirth.

RICHARDSON: *Well, my grandmother was kind of unusual. I understand that many midwives just disposed of it [the placenta] by burning. But my mother—my grandmother would bury hers. Uh-huhn. She would wrap it very, very neatly, and I would dig a hole, or whoever was there, the father, would dig a hole at a place where, you know, it could be watched and so on. They would put a stone or rock or a piece of tin or something over it. The hole would be deep enough where dogs couldn't get to it so easily, mm-hmm. She wasn't superstitious or anything like that, but she had a very sensitive nature about things like that being a part of a human being. She would always advise the father, whoever would bury it, to put it in a place where it was visible. That was a part of a person as far as she could see, and it was personally related.*

Like Richardson's grandmother, Lisa Weaver, the oldest known living lay midwife in Alabama at the time, knew about practices regarding burial of the placenta as well. Meeting Lisa Weaver days before she died at 110 was a reminder that women who supported her at the time of birthing could easily have been born during the era of enslavement. Holding in her hand a copy of the nursing home's newsletter that provided a snapshot of her legacy of decades of midwifery, Weaver spoke in whispers, but her eyes filled with the laughter that might have endeared her to mothers during the course of labor and birth. Weaver appeared to be a pillar of social support in her community.

Prior to our visiting Weaver, Taylor's "adopted mother," Taylor suggested taking a walk by Weaver's house, just blocks away from where Taylor lived. Walking past the pecan trees near the open gate to Weaver's front yard, I could see a yard filled with folks playing bid whist and jamming to soul music.

Noticing my surprise about the crowd gathered in the yard, Taylor for the first time referred to Weaver as Sister Scrapes.

> TAYLOR: *Sister could feed a whole bunch of children with-*
> *out having to go nowhere to borrow a cup of sugar or any-*
> *thing else. Folks knew if they had nowhere to stay, they*
> *could stay at Sister Scrapes's for days, months, years. She*
> *didn't know the word "no."*

Sister Scrapes died just weeks after I met her. When Taylor called to give me the news, she said, "You and me were the
last persons to visit her while she was still alive. You should
come to the funeral." That day folks leaned up against their cars
swapping Sister Scrapes stories in the Abraham Baptist Church
parking lot, creating the atmosphere of an outdoor wake. Once
we were inside the church, the elder deacon's opening prayer
made mention of how so few had gathered when there should
have been so many. When time came to make remarks, Taylor
was the only one who mentioned that Weaver waited on many
as a midwife. Speaking to the church congregation where folks
referred to each other as sisters and brothers, Taylor said, "Sister
was my second mother and trained me to be a midwife." Taylor
was the only one who remembered Weaver as their midwife,
so Taylor's tribute to the legendary midwife focused on how
Weaver cared for the entire community.

✳

Remembering Sister Scrapes's story reminds me how Penangnini Toure told me that his grandmother, Mama Aya, was a midwife who cared for her community in the Cote D'Ivoire where
he was born. Although Toure had described to his family how
respected his grandmother had been throughout the region,
he had never mentioned that she served the village as a midwife. Similar to Mama Scrapes in Montgomery, Mama Aya was
a holistic caregiver who, like so many midwives I met on the
Continent and in Alabama, had apprenticed with her mother.
    Growing up in a village where ancestors are viewed as the
intermediaries between living beings and God, Toure described

his grandmother's status and her extended role in his village of about 40 grass huts and 200 people. Speaking with reverence, Toure also referred to her knowledge in plant medicine and how she was respected not only in her village but by the people who traveled to the village from long distances seeking her advice. Like many midwives across the Continent, Toure's grandmother was a lineage midwife whose practices were rooted in timeless African beliefs and practices.

> TOURE: *She got it of course from her mother. You choose the person who is a wise person who could learn these secrets. In my community we are not Christians. We are not Muslims. We are farmers. Our ancestors are intermediaries between us living creatures, living beings and God. We consider our ancestors as saints. Talk to the ancestors. Ask for beneficiaries. Ask for the blessings of the gods. Ask for protection of the family. Men and women coming to see her for her wisdom. People coming from distant villages. She had status. People came to her to consult her. She was consulted like an elder, like a wise person. She was a doctor in that sense.*

And so was Mama Scrapes a caregiver whose hands touched the infants she cared for at birth and the adults whose lives she touched when they gathered to play bid whist in her yard. Toure and members of his village knew that the title "traditional birth attendant" failed to describe the scope and depth of Mama Aya's wisdom and service, just as folks at Mrs. Eliza Jane Weaver's funeral knew Weaver as a lifetime counselor. Toure explained that he named his daughter after his grandmother Aya, which means "born on Friday," because he believes his grandmother's wisdom lives in her.

CHAPTER 8

Lowndes County

Medicinal Herbs, Dirt Dauber Tea, Craving Earth

In 1981 the drive from Montgomery to Lowndesboro, Lowndes County, where I met Rosie Aaron Smith, an 85-year-old midwife, was supposed to take 30 minutes, but it always took me longer. Driving west on US 80 toward Selma, seeing the spirits of protestors beaten on Bloody Sunday rising up, always slowed me down. In 1965 state troopers had attacked civil rights activists peacefully walking across the then Pettus Bridge onto US 80 in a march to secure voting rights for Blacks. Days later, Viola Liuzzo was murdered on Highway 80 by the Ku Klux Klan as she shuttled activists leaving Selma to the Montgomery Airport on the now infamous highway.

Once I turned off US 80, my handwritten directions to Smith's house required looking out for groves of trees, a rural post office that looked like a painted white cottage, and counting the curves in the dirt road leading to the open area where there would be little to see other than the house where Smith lived. Smith later explained, "I pretty much built this house by myself except for the roof." The drive ended with my seeing Smith sitting barefoot on her front porch in a loosely fitting, plaid brown print dress with a hem lightly touching her sunscorched ankles.

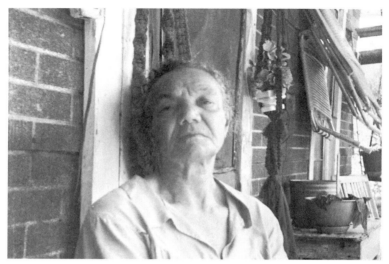

FIGURE 8.1. Rosie Aaron Smith sitting on her porch. Image permission by © Sharon Blackmon.

Like the midwives I met 40 years later on the Continent, Smith also was proud of her ability to care for herself and not be dependent on midwife assistance during labor and birth (see figure 8.1). Smith said, "I never laid around talking about what I can't do." Then added, "See the dress you have, I can make it. I just cut out the pattern in my mind." She also explained how she sometimes kept working through her labor pains before preparing to catch her own baby.

> SMITH: *I never hardly had no trouble with my pains. Most of the times, I had my babies before the midwife got there. And if I didn't beat the midwife to birthing, she wouldn't have much trouble. Oh, my babies would come out. Delivered all my babies pretty good. We would walk around as long as I felt good enough to walk around. Some of them I found them on the bed and some of them I found them on the floor. I just had a little pallet to go down on my knees . . .*
>
> *Sometimes I worked all day and [had] my baby that night. Now, I wasn't getting nervous unless it's right to the*

time. You know, you get real sick. Well, you would get a
little nervous, then you had to strain them nerves down.
Yeah, I worked. I never did quit working 'til I had my
babies. Well, I'd be at home doing my housework, you
know, piecing quilt or whatever I wanted to do.

There were times, however, that Smith did turn to the use of
plant medicines due to a problem that she called "female trouble": "Well, I don't know the name of the weed, but it was something that grows on the ground kind of like a little moss. Let
me see what we used to call it. We used to call it turkey weed."

Upon learning that turkey weed grew in the woods near
where she lived, Smith not only used the remedy herself but
recommended it to others. "'Course now, I didn't have no
license for that," Smith said. "But any lady could take care of a
lady to deliver a baby, she ought to be able to take care of her
with female trouble."

Smith first learned about turkey weed when meeting the
midwife who did "wait on her" in the past. At the time, Smith
was a tenant farmer and was sent to a white doctor by the white
landowner when sickness kept her from working. I'm not clear
what the medical diagnosis would be for what Smith described
as "female trouble," but she might have been diagnosed with
uterine prolapse (when the muscles and tissues of the pelvic
floor no longer provide adequate support for the uterus and
can cause the uterus to slip through the vagina). Mild cases
treated early may only require following recommended pelvic exercises. A lack of trust in her provider was her primary
concern.

SMITH: *And those doctors don't hardly do nothing for you.*
The doctors, they give you some kind of little tonic, and the
next thing, they want to operate on you for female trouble.
But now, oh Lord, I worked on so many people, female
trouble. Now, the ladies that I waited on, they hardly
would have much trouble with female troubles, but now

other ladies, I used to work on a lot of them for female trouble.

We used to call it turkey weed and you can get that turkey weed and boil it and give them that . . . I was still birthing my children at that time. And I suffered with my stomach a lot, and the doctor wanted to send me to the hospital. And I told him I wouldn't go.

So, time I got out the office, I met the lady that waited on me, the midwife lady, and I told her I was kind of weak. I said, "I been to the doctor now, Miss Emma." I said, "Could you help a lady with uh, female trouble?" She said, "Oh, honey, that's my occupation, delivering babies and lifting up the stomachs." I said, "Well, could I get you to help me?" I thought there was a big problem, you know. I said, "The doctor wanted me to go to the hospital."

She said, "I will work on you if you will wait and give me a trial." I said, "Well, I sure will because I ain't going to the hospital nohow."

That was on a Saturday.

I said, "Well, what should I do, Miss Emma? Would you come and stay with me two, three days and get me better, or would you want me to come and stay with you 'til I get better?"

She said, "Oh, no honey. There ain't no need of that. I will go and get my means together for what I need to work on you with and I'm going to tell you now how you use it."

Smith explained that her former midwife said, "I'm going to send you a tea. You drink that tea. Take a swallow or two of it anytime you feel like it." She said, "You ain't got to have no certain time. Two or three or four times, any time you feel like it, you take some of that tea." Smith replied, "Yes, ma'am," and thought, "I'm going to take it all the time."

SMITH: *So, I sent her two or three times for the tea, and I told her then I—my smartness came to me then. I said,*

"Miss Emma." She said, "Huh?" I said, "That stuff what you made me that tea out of," I said, "it's so far for me to send." I said, "Why don't you just send me some of the leaves and let me—I'll boil it like you say and make my own tea." She said, "Oh, well," she said, "I'll do that." When she sent the leaves, that put me on to what it was, you see. I said, "Oh, shucks." I said, these leaves grow right here. (laughter) The plants—these leaves grow out here [in our woods]. Anybody having trouble with their stomach then, just hunt for me. I wasn't a midwife then, still having babies myself. Until this day, if my children, you know, is having trouble with their stomach, they want to know, "Mama, can you find any of that vine that you used to make us that tea with?" (laughs) . . .

Once I had a cousin of mine come stay with me awhile a few years ago since I been here, and I found a little way down that hill in the woods there. But don't know if a lot of it grows around here. Where I used to live at, there would just be beds of it in the woods, and I was walking over it any time I went in the woods, but I didn't know what good it was.

While Smith indicated that the use of teas had pretty much faded out by the time she was having her babies, what she did remember stemmed mostly from the experience and advice she received from elders who continued to use plant-based medicines. In spite of separation from Mother Africa's rich ecology, Smith and other midwives across the diaspora succeeded in identifying plants in nearby forests and integrated their use into their midwifery practices. Unfortunately, harsh rules demanded that midwives abandon all use of plant medicines. Health department officials immediately revoked the license of any midwife known to incorporate the use of plant-based medicine or teas in their practice. Like midwives I met on the Continent, however, Smith viewed childbirth as an experience she could manage independently.

Years later, when Smith's daughter decided to give birth in her mother's home, Smith said, "I saw I could do for my daughter what the midwife did for me." In 1948 Smith, who had only a sixth-grade education but years of what she proudly called fireside learning from her grandmother, began practicing as a licensed lay midwife in Lowndes County.

Mary Aaron, who apprenticed with Smith decades later, was among the last generation of Black lay midwives to obtain a permit to practice in Alabama. Acquiring her midwife permit at the age of 21, Aaron lived in Lowndesboro when she was having her babies, and Smith was her midwife. In Lowndes County, nurses recruited younger women to become midwives who would then need to pass a written test followed by an apprenticeship that required attending at least three births. Health department rules prohibited the use of plant-based medicine, similar to the restrictions TBAs described 40 years later in Kpana Village and in Ejura in Ghana. The Alabama Health Department process for becoming a lay midwife differed from the traditional way on the Continent, where senior midwives often determined the qualities, skills, and sensibilities needed to assist mothers at birth. There, a respected community-based midwife often chose a family member or a person she observed having the potential to continue her midwife practice when she retired and asked her to begin assisting them at births and in apprenticeships of varying lengths. About why the nurse selected her for midwife training, Aaron said, "She saw how clean and neatly dressed I was, and she decided I would make a good midwife."

AARON: *A white nurse used to come and make home visits. My uncle was sick with tuberculosis and had to get shots. Whenever I knew she was coming, I would change and look nice. So, the nurse noticed how neat and clean I was dressed. Then one day the nurse said, "Would you like to be a midwife?" She said, "Mrs. Aaron, you're always so clean when we come." Said, "You would just make a nice midwife," she said, just out of the blue. I said, "Oh, fine,*

I'd just love it," not even knowing really what it was. And that's just how I got started really. I really didn't know what I was getting into. I just said "yes."

The training was up at the Health Department in Lowndes County. We would go to a meeting every first and third Wednesday, and then they would assign you to a licensed midwife. And then you were given a great big manual to study, and then you went over all these questions and everything. And when you finished, they would always ask you "Are you ready for your test?" So, then I said "Not yet." And I was really afraid to take it, you know. So finally I said, "I think I'm ready."

And then, you know, it was Miss Rosie Aaron Smith—she was the midwife who delivered all my babies—I was assigned to her. She was really kind of helpful because she would let me do a lot of things and then she'd say, "Do you think you could do this?" And then finally they asked me, did I think I was ready to go out on my own, and I told them, I really believed I could do it.

While Aaron said she learned from her training to never use herbal medicines of any kind in her practice as a lay midwife, she vividly remembered women who gathered to support her when she was giving birth telling her to drink dirt dauber tea, which is made from a dirt dauber's nest. While nature controls most aspects of labor and birth for most mothers, there can be complications. Medical practitioners in hospital settings may use the drug Pitocin to induce labor when there are concerns that the health of the mother or baby may be at risk. In the 1970s, however, women's groups began to vehemently object to the inappropriate use and overuse of drugs such as Pitocin because of possible side effects.

Similar to midwives on the Continent, Aaron also described how women gathered to support mothers during labor and birth. Women celebrated with chanting and praise in villages in Kenya and with ululations and coffee ceremonies in Ethiopia.

When Aaron gave birth in Lowndesboro, she said, "the room would be so full of women—sometimes ten women—in and out." Even though Aaron was dismissive of teas made from dirt dauber's nests or black pepper tea, which midwives described as effective in promoting labor, she acknowledged that there might be some efficacy in the teas based on her personal experience.

> AARON: Listen, honey. When I had my babies, they had— these old women—they gave me dirt dauber tea and they gave me castor oil. If I wasn't having pains like they thought that I should have. So Ms. Aaron [Rosie Aaron Smith] said, "I'm tired of sitting here. I'm ready to go home." She would get some of that hot pepper and that just plain old dirt.
>
> You know anything about dirt daubers? A dirt dauber looks like a wasp, a yellow jack[et]. Okay, they build these nests and it's made out of mud, just plain mud. So they would get two or three of them old mud nests and put it in water and get some red, just plain red pepper that grow in the field, the field you know, and put it in there and boil it, and they let me drink it just as hot as I can bear it. Lord! And I would just drink it. And really, I don't know if it was a psychological thing, that it seemed like the pains would just start coming, and they would just come.
>
> And they would give ginger tea sometime. They would give this hot ginger tea. And we would take that stuff. Just put the dirt in there and put some water on it and then— break up the pepper in there, and then let it boil. Just steep, steep it. You know they wouldn't let the dirt fall in there. Just the muddiest looking water. And I would drink that. Yeah, she stayed there as long as she could. Then she'd say, "I'm tired now, and I'm going on and get through with it." And she'd give me that tea. And, honey, I'm telling you the truth—Yes sir. I guess—I mean, I felt like it helped.

Jennie Rawlinson, a retired midwife who lived in neighboring Autauga County, was so committed to the use of dirt dauber tea that she continued making the tea for her daughters even when they were having their babies in the hospital.

> RAWLINSON: *I didn't deliver my children—the babies—but when they got in labor, they would come, you know, and they didn't want to go to the hospital too early and things like that, so I gave mine some dirt dauber tea. I tied it up into a thin piece and put it in water and let it boil. And I would take another thin piece and strain it. Steep a little bit, Mm-mm. It's kind of like muddy water. It makes those pains come. They started coming pretty regular. We take it and then go to the hospital. Mm-hmm, yeah.*

Midwives in Alabama who learned about the making of dirt dauber tea from elders in their families had no way of knowing that dirt dauber beverages had been used by midwives and healers on the Continent since the beginning of time. Unfortunately, many academic studies have dismissed the eating of any type of clay as not having benefits that could be documented by scientific research. Scientists in Zimbabwe are challenging this view, finding chemicals in the dirt used to make dirt dauber tea that are similar to oxytocin, a hormone that sends a chemical message from the brain that initiates labor contractions.

In addition to drinking dirt dauber tea, pregnant women in the United States and in West Africa are also known for craving earth to eat during pregnancy, which is known as geophagy. In the US, the practice was thought to be a southern phenomenon and was often attributed to ignorance or hunger; after the Great Migration to urban cities, health care providers became aware of pregnant women having white and red clay shipped to them because they couldn't find the quality of clay they were seeking in northern cities. When women were unable to obtain the earth they craved, eating starch became a substitute. Unfortunately, starch lacks any of the essential minerals like magnesium, phosphorus, potassium, and zinc that researchers are finding in their analysis of the earth that women crave during pregnancy in Ghana.

In Alabama and on the Continent, I met women who were selective in choosing the type of earth they craved during pregnancy. A midwife in Ethiopia explained that the mothers she knew wanted to consume only a special type of black earth that was sold in a marketplace in a nearby village. In Alabama, one midwife kept secret the location of a red dirt mound because she had made a business of shipping selected earth to pregnant women living in New York. Another midwife I met baked white clay in her oven for me to sample because she believed her clay had an irresistible cheeselike flavor that I would enjoy. And I did.

For Lula Holiday, however, earth eating had spiritual significance.

> HOLIDAY: I craved dirt. I had to eat dirt sometime too. It looked like it tasted better than anything. And, you know, it's back to the dust we must go. We all got to eat so much dust or dirt or something or other. I just crave it at times. I don't know why. At times, it would be better to me than my food. It just looked like I had to have some dirt. I think it is more spiritual 'cause it says back to the dust you must go. You gotta have so much dust or dirt in your body. And God said you gotta go back there. You got to have it in your body to go back. It's just a spiritual thing. That's natural. Sometimes when it was muddy, I'd just put it in the stove and just dry it and bake it or something, and it look like it would taste better.

Midwives and healers on the Continent have used selected earth in their pharmacopeia from time immemorial, and scientists in Ghana are finding differences in the chemical makeup of selected samples of earth that women were known to crave during pregnancy. For example, midwives have their ways of knowing that kaolin found in white clay is an effective treatment for diarrhea and is sometimes applied to wounds to stop bleeding. Reds soils appear to be rich in iron.

Enslaved Africans might have heard creation stories from their ancestors that included dirt daubers, like those that begin with how God first created "the earth from soft mud." Unlike in the Old Testament where God creates man and woman first, in this West African creation story, first the chameleon, the water, and the fish are created, and then the cat, the dog, the toad, and the mud dauber wasp. The story ends with God creating man and woman. When gathering earth from a dirt dauber's nest to make tea for a mother preparing to give birth, could the great-grandmothers of Black midwives I met in Alabama have seen dirt daubers not just as insects but as a part of traditional African creation stories?

Similar to midwives on the Continent, Lowndes County midwives were consulted when seeking remedies for general sicknesses as well as for herbal medicines during pregnancy, labor, and birth. Smith, for example, recalled elders using jimson weed to make a tea to treat fevers. "They'd get them jimson weeds and boil them and let that tea get cold, cool, and they'd bathe you with them," Smith said. "It was real good for fever. It'll help you."

Pinkey Nix, a midwife who also practiced in Lowndes County, recommended using tread sash to make a necklace to tie around an infant's neck as a treatment for fever.

> NIX: Well, to tell you the truth—now if they got a high fever, you give them old tread sash. They string it around the baby's neck. That cools that fever right down . . . You just dig it [tread sash] up. Then you get a root, a white root. It's about the size of a match, and you get those roots and you clean them off and you take a knife and cut around, just strip it off, and leave the hard stem inside. Then you thread them and put them round the neck like a necklace. It don't smell good, but it sure takes the fever. Just put it around there green.

Remembering how elders in her family combined quinine with fresh lard that was mixed into a salve to "rub you all over with" as a way to reduce fever, midwife Alberta Motley described how the elders she knew recommended that women find a "big old collard leaf or just mostly any kind of big wide leaf like a mullet when suffering with a fever."

MOTLEY: *Have you seen a big old leaf growing out in the woods that looks like a cabbage? That's how a mullet leaf looks.*

The practice of wrapping heated green leaves from specific plants around your head when suffering with a headache continues in parts of Jamaica. An image, housed at the North Carolina Museum of History, of an enslaved women with a large collard green around her head in North Carolina, is an indication that the tradition of green-leaf head wrapping for a headache may be widespread among women of African descent.

While practices among midwives in Lowndes County were remembered by elders, the 1976 law eliminating midwives ended the passing of herbal knowledge on to their daughters, granddaughters, or whoever they may have chosen to continue their practices. Midwives on the Continent continued to refresh their knowledge by returning home to their village, where elders whose knowledge regarding preparing medicines made from plants, seeds, and bark used in childbirth distinguished them.

For example, Naomi, a midwife who lived in a Nairobi settlement, described her frequent visits back to the village where she benefited from watching her mother make the teas and medicines that she initially learned from her. By 1981 the former midwives in Alabama had only memories of elders in their families seeking out their grandmothers in rural areas who knew how to go to the woods and identify herbs for healing, just as Naomi described.

NAOMI: *When I go back to the village, I know what I am*

looking for. I know the leaves. I used to ask my mother whenever I came about herbs used for the mother for cleansing after birth, herbs to help mothers who can't conceive, and herbs to help the infant to grow. There is medicine which if someone is bleeding, it stops the bleeding. It is herbal. I boil it. It is for drinking. It is traditional. It just grows, so I go to look for it knowing what I am looking for. Before leaving home, I asked my mother about medicine that can cure a particular thing and she tells me it is this. There is one for boiling and there is one that is just put in water and she drinks it cold to stop the bleeding.

Alabama midwives also knew what they were looking for when searching for plants in the woods or growing herbs in their gardens, even after the state dismantled the system of experienced midwives passing their knowledge down to younger midwives. Even so, I sensed that I was a "daughter" that Smith chose to pass her stories on to.

Smith continued her midwife practice until 1967, two years after Viola Liuzzo was murdered in Lowndesboro just a few miles away from where Smith lived. Ku Klux Klan members shot Liuzzo as she was driving Black civil rights activists back to the Montgomery Airport from Selma after the historic voters' rights march over the Edmund Pettus Bridge. Smith recalled the impact of the civil rights movement and the march that became known as Bloody Sunday.

SMITH: *I wasn't involved, but you see, white people mostly got against most all colored folks about that. They got against all colored people. White people had the people kind of like slaves. I used to live down in the bottom. I moved when the civil rights movement came through. They didn't want colored on the land. White people wouldn't rent the colored people their land to farm on it. They'd just rather let it grow up and put cows on it, let trees grow up on it. You just couldn't hardly get grocery without the white man letting you have it. And everything you made on his land, it had to go through his hands mostly. Would let you have only what he wanted you to have.*

Similar to midwives on the Continent, Smith didn't view her services as a midwife as a money-generating business. Referring to how the Alabama Health Department established the fees that midwives should charge, Smith again asserted her independence.

SMITH: *The law put a price on us for us to charge for people. That's the only way I would charge that much, and sometimes I wouldn't charge them that much; I would, you know, take less than that . . . I thought it was nice to do some good for somebody that needed good, I always thought. That's why I never was so hard on people about the money. I always done it in the name of the Lord, to help somebody.*

[I would tell them] "Now, don't tell everybody." I said, "'Cause the law is so much." Well, before I quit being a midwife, the law had worked us up from $5 to $10, from $10 to $15. Now, they had got up—just before I quit, they had started asking for $20 or $25, one. It was either $20 or $25, but I know they worked them up $5 at a time. They would say they didn't know how we could work, you know, for people and wait on people for that little money. I could wait on them 'cause I worked in the fields for my living, but oh, that was a help, you know. Yeah, that was a help—and love to do good things in the name of the Lord. I always thought the Lord was a good-paying man.

Now, some people were pretty good about paying you and some people wouldn't pay you on time. (laughs) Some people owe me—Lord, if I had the money people owed me now, I could be living comfortable. Because some people I waited on, I didn't never get a dime from. Some of them I waited on a second time and didn't get paid . . . I had a

Christian heart about that. If you didn't have nothing, I didn't want nothing. I figured if they had the right kind of heart, when they'd get something, they would give me something.

As regulations governing midwife practices continued to escalate, Smith, who trusted her experiences and lessons learned from elders in the community, chose to retire. A decade before the state of Alabama decided to eliminate issuing lay-midwife permits, Smith decided to end her practice as a midwife, as the uncertainties of the impact of the historic civil rights and Black Power movements swirled around her in Lowndes County.

> SMITH: *When the nurse wrote it up on the board in the office that Rosie was no more a midwife, she said people said, "Oh, what are we going to do now?" I told her they'd just have to find themselves somebody else because she had to give up to take care of her own people at home. Oh, the county went into mourning; when I gave up my license of being a midwife, the county went into mourning. The nurse told me, when I went back again, "Rosie, I never had such a crying as I had when you said you would no more be a midwife."*

From the era of enslavement until the 1960s, the culture of white supremacy and Jim Crow shut most Black women and their families in Lowndes County and across Alabama out of mainstream health care. Even when access to white doctors increased, Black families exercised their privilege to reject medical care from white doctors because of mistrust and mistreatment. When Smith had a choice between surgery with a doctor for her female troubles and using an herbal recommended by an older midwife, she chose turkey weed tea as her midwife advised. "We didn't have all kinds of sickness like we have now," Smith said. "We had that good feed."

CHAPTER 9

Selma, Dallas County

Outdooring Ceremony, Keeping a Birth Fire, Elements of Protection

Selma, Dallas County, will always be my Alabama home. I went to Selma for the first time in 1971 to visit a college friend whose family was on the front lines of Selma's civil rights movement. Leola Robertson, my classmate's mother, housed and fed countless SNCC (Student Nonviolent Coordinating Committee) workers in the early days of the youth-led movement. On September 15, 1963, the day after the bombing of the Birmingham church that killed four Black girls, Robertson's oldest son, Willie C., was beaten in the head by the owner of Carter Drug Store for wanting to be served at the drug store counter. Willie C.'s refusal to bow down to Jim Crow laws was among the pivotal acts that sparked the Selma civil rights movement for justice.

I met midwives in Selma and other Black Belt communities who described how their ancestors managed to support traditions and create environments that fostered rest and renewal during the vulnerable weeks following birth. Robertson said that her grandmother, who was the midwife "for just about everybody in the family," inspired her to become a nurse and to keep her home open for SNCC workers to stay during the height of the movement. When she opened her door to young SNCC workers in the '60s, Robertson said that she was emulating her grandmother's caring ways—she had witnessed her grandmother feeding and sheltering women in her family during birth and the weeks that followed.

I met midwives on the Continent who remembered culturally based practices supported by midwives in their villages such as naming ceremonies, smoking the mother, and keeping a birth fire continuously burning for weeks. In Alabama, Black midwives described similar practices and referred to them as following the old rules or keeping the ways of the elders. At the time, no one suggested that these practices reflected their African heritage, but I now know that they did. I can clearly see within the rituals of midwives of African descent expressions of religious beliefs, such as seeing the return of an ancestor in the birth of a baby.

While Alabama midwives during enslavement through the Jim Crow era had few opportunities to communicate with each other, they sustained similar birthing traditions and beliefs, all of which reflected how women supported women at birth. The survival of these traditions into the 1970s is a tribute to the strength and determination of Black women to keep these practices alive.

In Selma I met Rosie Price, a midwife who remembered the stories of the "slave time people" in her family. Price described the hardships of enslavement, as told by her family elders, who remembered the adversities. No one in her family had been a midwife, but she followed the traditions of birthing rituals passed down to her from elders of her family for generations.

PRICE: *My mother's mother died when she was a small girl. Only thing I know on my mother's side was her uncle and her aunt, and my great-grandmother. I was a small girl, but I do remember them. I have heard my great-grandmother say that her mother brought her here from Africa. She said she was a small girl and those other kids, other girls, were older than she was. I'm thinking that she was the baby or next to the baby . . . Yeah. She said at that time that they couldn't go to church. They couldn't pray. If the master heard you praying, he'll whip the Devil out ya. You know, that was rough then. He didn't do a thing but just make 'em stay out there and work all the time, and if he had a good woman, she was a breeder. He let her stay at the house and do the cooking and do the breeding.*

Price described her working conditions that continued throughout her pregnancy and the traditions she adhered to following birth.

PRICE: We just want a big crop, because we had a lot of children . . . You had to have a big crop to pay your debt out and then sometimes you couldn't pay it out . . . You see, we would have so much of it in corn, so much of it in peas, so much in potato, and so much in cotton.

Picking cotton. Picking cotton, breaking corn, digging potatoes and peanuts and so forth. Just on a big farm. Me and my husband and my children. I could pick 200 pounds of cotton. He'd pick 300 pounds and we would just get on out there and just get to work. Oh, boy. Well, that's the way we worked. But you had to have a big farm to try to make all you could. We was working for ourselves, but we had to pay rent. We had to pay that. And see, you had to have enough to work at just to pay those debts out.

In the midst of demeaning systems of tenant farming and sharecropping, Price and other mothers honored what they viewed as the "old-time ways" when they adhered to the postpartum birthing traditions, including that one of the places women could make a way to reinforce their own cultural practices and traditions was in sustaining traditions surrounding birth.

In Africa, birthing was a time for ceremony and ritual celebrated in seeing the return of an ancestor in the spirit of the newborn. Price preserved rituals that recognized both seeing the spirit of the baby and caring for the infant's physical needs.

Her ancestors had also preserved portions of the more elaborate naming ceremonies practiced on the Continent.

Another retired Selma midwife, Ollie Burns, who described the traditions surrounding birth promulgated by the elder midwives as "something we used to do," remembered elders telling her not to extinguish the fire that was burning at the time of birth and to wait a month or even longer before sweeping the birth fire ashes outside of the house. Burns said, "You could sweep 'em back, but you couldn't take 'em up." With laughter, Burns recalled postpartum rules that included bringing a thimble of water back from the spring for the baby when going outdoors for the first time; she honored them. "Yeah, when I had my first, they made me go around the house nine times. Just walk around the house, carrying the baby," Burns said. "And I never knew what all that was supposed to have been for."

For Cora Bell Marshall, a retired midwife I also met in Selma, traditions surrounding birth were simply known as "the old-time business." Marshall was called to take up her mother's midwifery practice when her mother became ill. Initially, Marshall practiced as an unlicensed midwife under the supervision of a white doctor. "I delivered the baby," Marshall said. "The doctor wasn't there. He got paid $10 and he gave me $2 or $3." Marshall eventually became a licensed lay midwife and practiced independently. Although she eventually rejected the rituals that lost meaning for her, Marshall remembered the details she once followed in the ritual, recognizing the importance of seeing and calling the "spirit" of the baby. Marshall and others referred to this ritual as the "outdooring" after birth.

> MARSHALL: *I ain't forgot that [outdooring]. They always say, "Call the baby. When you walk out the door, call the baby." I call him, "MC come on. MC, come on" . . . Then she would say, "You ain't calling this boy." I'd call him again. I called him until I got back in the house. Now what good did that do? (laughing) . . .*

She just told me, "Yes. Yes," that is what she said. "Call that baby's Spirit."

That was the old-time way. She certainly sure did throw a cover over my head, and she'd tote the baby and told me to call that baby. See, I was calling his spirit—calling that baby's name and all the way around the house she says, "You ain't calling this boy." Come on and I'd say it again and come on back in the house and I'd sit down.

That's olden-time business. I went out this way and went around the house with something over my coat and went all around and come on back and come in the house. I sure did that. That's old times. I did that about three times with my babies, but the rest of them I had gotten on the fast pace. I didn't do that anymore.

While in Kenya, Ethiopia, and Ghana, I learned how mid-wives described postpartum birthing traditions in terms that reflected a traditional African religion or their Islamic faith. In Alabama, however, the midwives and elders I met described their "outdooring" rituals in words that reflected their faith in Jesus. When Alabama midwives instructed mothers to call the baby's spirit before going back indoors, they might suggest praying in the name of Jesus. Midwives I met in Alabama and on the Continent agreed that the newborn's spirit remained in both earthly and spiritual realms and could easily return to the world of the deities.

Rituals and ceremonies that were part of the postpartum regimen also protected the mother. Although not mentioned as often as the outdooring ceremony of circling the house and calling the baby's spirit, another tradition that paralleled practices on the Continent was "smoking the mother," as part of the first outdooring ritual. Thelma Shamburger, who worked in the Black Belt before later practicing as a midwife in Mobile, Alabama, described the practice she observed in Wilcox County. "First the mother circled the house," Shamburger said. "Then they'll smoke them—put the smoke on her." She laughed. "I don't know what there'd be in that paper."

Raised by her grandmother, who was born in Africa, Margaret Charles Smith, a midwife who attended thousands, provided more details about the ritual she observed from having watched her grandmother smoke her clothes and undergarments before going outdoors for the first time after childbirth. Living in Eutaw, Greene County, Alabama, Smith explained that her grandmother added cornmeal to the fireplace fire before the garments were passed through the smoke in this ritual of purification. The time following birth was viewed as particularly vulnerable. The use of cornmeal in "smoking the mother" may have been influenced by local Native American traditions where cornmeal is used in sacred ceremonies.

In Marian, 30 miles south of Selma, Mary Martin, a third-generation midwife in her 70s, remembered her grandmother "smoking the mother" as well. Martin said, "My grandmother used to go back and take 'em up, and that ritual was part of the 'taking up' practice." She said, "But I ain't never took 'em up now."

On the Continent, midwives described other rituals that served to reduce anxiety and stress by assuring the mother that she was protected and could rest in the weeks following labor and birth. In Ghana, midwives I met described the practice of placing herbs into the fire to "smoke the mother" in order to drive bad spirits away. For example, I met a midwife in Kpana who described, how Tikuhum, an herbal medicine, is added to the fire to protect the child or mother from evil spirits. These herbs may have also had a calming psychological effect.

Following "outdooring" ceremonies on the Continent, the time for seclusion and purification was 40 days in Islamic communities and sometimes as long as two months in villages adhering to traditional African practices. In Alabama, midwives described how during the postpartum period, mothers rested while other women—often the mother, mother-in-law, or midwife—made certain that the birth fire was never extinguished, ashes were swept away at the appropriate time, and food was prepared for the mother and her family members.

Midwives in Alabama also remembered forks, scissors, axes, or other items containing metals being placed under the mattress to "cut" afterbirth pain and to promote healing in the postpartum period. On the Continent, metals also are used for medicinal purposes and protection. Among the Yoruba, for example, iron, the symbol for Ogun, is one of the religion's most powerful deities. In Kenya, blacksmiths make protective amulets from iron for placing at altars or in sacred gardens. And in Kenya, the metal knife used to cut the umbilical cord may be placed under the baby's pillow to protect the child from harm by evil spirits.

Mary Smith, one of the last midwives I met in Selma, knew about traditions as the mother of 16 children, including two children, about whom Smith said, "them, I delivered myself." Smith was among the younger midwives who questioned the validity of the rules that her mother-in-law wanted her to follow, but she appreciated the support and care she received from her mother and her sister during the postpartum period, which included cooking food for the family and caring for the children. Smith was well informed about a range of postpartum practices, which included using metals for healing. In recalling birthing traditions, Smith punctuated her stories with good humor and outbursts of laughter.

> SMITH: *You know what the older mothers used to do? Used to take forks and put 'em up under the bed. They would take forks and cross 'em up and put them under the mother's bed, and they always said they'd slip them under there and the mother wouldn't know they were under the mattress. And that would cut off some of that pain. And oh, they said you couldn't sweep out under your bed. You know my mother-in-law and my husband or the midwife could sweep under my bed, but said I couldn't sweep out from under there until the baby's at least a month old. I*

followed that. But all these others, I haven't paid that any attention.

You know, we used to have a fireplace, and they wouldn't let you carry any ashes out until the baby was a month old. I don't know what that was supposed to have been. They say you're carrying the life of the baby, the breath or something. Yeah, and they didn't allow you to cook. They said that the mother wasn't clean yet. Mm-hmm. You know when you have a baby you just kind of have a fresh scent, you know, that I don't care how you bathe yourself, it's just something about that baby that kind of stays with you for a while. And I think they felt like the mother was never clean enough to be around food, so they always prepared it and brought it to me. My mother-in-law did that 'til my baby got four weeks old. She wanted me to eat chicken, rice, eggs, and maybe . . . No, even no milk. She didn't want me to have milk.

But I ate, I tell you what! My husband, he had been fishing, and so he got out there and cleaned the fish. My baby was four weeks old now, and they said you couldn't eat fish 'til the baby was six weeks old. We couldn't have fish and no wild food—stuff like rabbits and goats and fish, stuff like that. They said you couldn't have it. And she asked me would it give me a headache to fry fish. I said, "No." And she fried that fish and I had so much I was drunk. (laughter)

The fish didn't do anything, but all that grease, you know, and I'm trying to eat a lot of fish before they catch me, and if I hadn't of burnt the bottom, they wouldn't have. I ate so much fish, and she said, "Lord, I hope you don't die, 'cause if you do your mother will swear I killed you!" (laughter)

But it didn't do anything to me. But I mean chicken and chicken and chicken. That's all she wanted me to eat in the meat line. I could eat eggs, she said. I was staying with my mother-in-law, yeah. And grits and rice, all the grits and rice you wanted. And I mean for dinner you had to have a little bowls of rice and some chicken. And people didn't have refrigerators and things like they do now, and she would cut up that chicken, and we go out and catch them out in the yard, and she cut up one, and she just cooked that chicken for me, 'cause she cooking maybe like sausage and stuff for my husband and herself . . .

And I always was taught you couldn't have sex until the baby was six weeks old. Well, I tell you what—he didn't. My first child he didn't 'cause we had two beds. After then we had to after so many babies, the beds got so full, he had no other choice (laughter) but to sleep in the bed with me. But I was always taught you couldn't have sex until the baby was six weeks old.

Now, on the Continent, some of the younger TBAs I met also questioned some of the food restrictions passed on to them by senior traditional midwives in their communities. In Alabama, several midwives I interviewed in the 1980s agreed that they continued to follow birthing traditions that had no social, psychological, or spiritual significance for them out of respect for their grandmothers or other family elders. Now some of the younger midwives I met on the Continent are part of a growing movement to assert the rights of women to reject aspects of traditional birthing culture, particularly rules that restrict women to mothering roles or that fail to recognize the right of mothers to decide what kinds of rituals or other traditions they want to include in their birth experience.

Mama Adzorhlor III, born in the village of Dagbamete in Ghana and now living in Canada, is a young botanist who continues to immerse herself in the traditional ways of her grandmother, Adzorhlor Davor, a midwife in her community for more than 50 years. "My grandmother must be close to a hundred," Adzorhlor told me in a telephone interview in 2021. "But whenever I ask my grandmother to tell me her age, she just laughs and says, 'I'm 170 years old!'"

Adzorhlor's grandmother's ways of assisting mothers and babies included herbal baths, massages, protective rituals, and extending spiritual blessings that ward off evil spirits. "Our village is surrounded by forests. Our ancestors understood that mothers and babies may have weakened immune systems requiring extra protection."

> ADZORHLOR: *Being indoors, the mother feels safe, and she can get her energy back. A lot can happen in the days immediately following birth, so it was important to hold and protect the mother and the baby. That was the task of the grandmother. They did not let everyone visit, just the people in your bubble, as we say now. They were the only ones having access.*
>
> *My grandmother went to a training program, and she could not believe that the guidelines in the training said that they wanted all mothers to lie down in bed when having their babies! The trainings emphasize only book learning. My grandmother's wisdom deserves respect as well.*

After watching her grandmother attending a birth in her village, Adzorhlor said, "I could see the energy and strength flowing from her eyes, connecting with the mother." She continued, "It's unbelievable—watching the energy flow between them. Seeing my grandmother in that way gave me strength to have my children at home."

In Selma, even though it was years after her grandmother's death, Robertson also deeply respected how her grandmother upheld birthing traditions and created environments that fostered renewal in the time following birth in spite of the stress that Black women encountered in Jim Crow Alabama. Robertson's first baby was also born at home with a midwife who wanted her to respect birthing traditions.

> ROBERTSON: *My grandmother reared me. My mother died when I was 12. She always did for others. My grandmother*

*was the one just taking care of her family. She was the mid-
wife for all her children. We called her Mama. I think my
grandmother was my mother's midwife . . .*

*My grandmother didn't care if she got paid or not; she
would go. She didn't care how it rained; she would go. My
grandmother rode mules and buggies and nearly froze to
death.*

When Leola Robertson had her babies, her grandmother
was no longer living, but the traditional tapestry surrounding
birth was a shared one. How Robertson described her birthing experience is similar to what most Black midwives simply
defined as "the old-time way."

ROBERTSON: *Elnora Houston, who waited on me, was
really good because she said I could eat anything. But that
month was puzzling. Wouldn't allow you to wash your
hair. I just couldn't wait for my month to be up so I could
go to the beautician.*

*In those days men didn't like to eat women's cooking
when they had babies. When your womb is still open, you
are not supposed to be around men.*

*And you couldn't take ashes out for a month. I imag-
ine everything isn't burned out. They want everything
kept inside until they take you out. Maybe something
could happen. If somebody was against you, they could
do something. I was told to be careful. From those ashes
they could be in touch with your body. I was just so
worried.*

*When the month was up, take the baby, go all the way
around the house. I did that with Willie C., my first baby.
You do whatever you think you want to do, like sing or
talk. I carried the baby. The midwife went around because
she figured I would be weak. She said I could sing. I think
the song I sang—yes, I know the song I sang. It was "Jesus
Is All to Me." Yes, that was the song . . .*

> *I liked the midwife better than a doctor. Miss Elnora checked on me at least twice a month, and she came back to see me after the baby was born. She was really nice. A lot of times she would bring me food. She was really a sweet nurse, just like my grandmother.*
>
> *See, a midwife takes more time. When you are having your baby, the midwife talks to you. I could hear her praying when I was in labor. I could hear her saying "Lord have mercy." But you know what the doctor did? He just said, "Go ahead and have your baby."*

Despite the gains of the civil rights movement, 20 years after the Selma to Montgomery march, when I was conducting these interviews in Alabama, dehumanizing practices continued to mark medical care in Selma. Even though the Jim Crow signs had come down, there were still separate waiting rooms for Black and white patients. Black women in Alabama also told me about white doctors who would see Black patients on days and times that were different from when they saw white patients. Dr. Jessee Howard said that when he decided to open his practice in Dallas County in 1980, "a white doctor who had her office enclosed in a fence would come out in the morning and pass out 40 tickets through the fence. Whatever 40 people got there first, that's who she would see."

When Dr. Howard opened up his office, which included an out-of-hospital birthing suite, he hired Mary Aaron, a lay midwife I interviewed in Lowndes County who apprenticed with Rosie Aaron Smith. Aaron said, "You know, I was on call for Dr. Jesse Howard down in Selma for one year from 6:00 at night until 6:00 in the morning."

Howard was impressed with Aaron's skills and the skills of midwives he observed when pursuing his medical degree at Tuskegee University. "I don't remember having to repair a perineal tear that happened in a midwife delivery," Howard said, remembering how midwives cared for mothers at Tuskegee's hospital. "Yeah, they called them granny midwives, but they really were the doctors. They had to be because they couldn't get to a doctor or hospital for back-up. I learned from them." Howard also knew Ella Foster, his mother's midwife. Howard said, with pride, "A midwife delivered me and 11 of my siblings."

In 1963, when activists marched from Selma to Montgomery demanding civil rights and justice, they walked the same road that enslaved Africans struggled to survive on during the journey to Dallas County after being sold on Montgomery's auction block, one of the most lucrative auction blocks in the Deep South. Black activists, like Willie C. Robertson, whose great-grandmother was a midwife, knew that a "midwife got him here." For generations, Black midwives managed to create and shelter birthing spaces that did not crumble under the medical mockery and degradation that public health officials threatened them with.

CHAPTER 10

Mobile and Beyond

Advisors, Advocates, Lifetime Caregivers

Mobile, Alabama, is the only place in the United States where it is possible to document an African American midwife's extended role in a Black community that was established by the last enslaved Africans transported across the Atlantic from the Continent. This is because in 1860 Timothy Meaher, a wealthy Mobile plantation owner, defied international law and smuggled 110 young adults and children into Mobile 52 years after transatlantic slave trade was outlawed.

Following Emancipation, some of the Yoruba-speaking Africans who could not raise the money needed to return to their homeland purchased small plots of land from the plantation owner who had previously enslaved them. Three miles north of downtown Mobile, the founders of Africatown—also known as Plateau—established an independent Black community that grew to include a church, a community burial ground, small Black-owned businesses, and a school housed in the Union Baptist Church. Championed by Booker T. Washington, the school became the oldest Rosenwald School in continuous use in the nation. Africatown also became a safe haven for preserving traditions such as keeping Yoruba names and continuing the Ikomajade naming ceremony translated as "giving the child a crown," as described by Natalie S. Robertson in *The Slave Ship*

Clotilda and the Making of AfricaTown, USA. Use of herbal medicines, support for home birth, and preference for midwives as holistic caregivers remained an uninterrupted tradition in Africatown throughout the 1970s. In 2019 UNESCO recognized Africatown as a site of memory in its international "Slave Route Project: Resistance, Liberty, Heritage."

Mobile is also the only place in Alabama where I returned to interview midwife descendants and community members after my travel to Africa. Returning to Africatown for the first time in September 2019, 38 years after first meeting Thelma Shamburger, a renowned Mobile midwife, I wanted to see if the house where I met her was still standing. Not only was Shamburger's house decimated, Shamburger's historic neighborhood looked like it could have been bombed. The vibrant community where I met Shamburger in 1981 was no longer on the map.

Even though forty years ago, I rarely used a map. I was accustomed to directions that described curves in the roads and clusters of oak trees adorned with moss and that ended with looking out for a midwife who said she would be sitting on her front porch shelling peas. Shamburger, the midwife I interviewed in Africatown, advised looking out for industrial landmarks like the International Paper Company, which I later learned was built on land owned by the same Meaher family that had enslaved the Africans on their plantation. Driving past the smokestacks that polluted the air several times, I knew I was lost.

Seeing a mailman, I pulled over and asked for help.

"I am trying to find Mrs. Thelma Shamburger," I said, showing him the paper with Front Street scribbled on it with no specific address.

"Oh, you mean Mama Thelma, the midwife. She lives in the yellow house not too far from here."

His directions got me there in minutes.

I met Shamburger standing barefoot on the front porch of her home, next door to the house where she was born. "They keep changing the name of the street," Shamburger said, "but I was born right next door. I have never moved since I was born, just from that house to over here."

Wearing a white housecoat with red polka dots, Shamburger, 70 years old, welcomed me into her house filled with piles of books and baskets of home remedies as she began to explain how she happened to attend her first birth in Wilcox County. Shamburger kept an open door, making it easy for neighbors and even one of the children she delivered to drop in and out of our conversation. Looking over her spectacles with one temple piece missing, Shamburger kept an eye on welcoming visitors, who sometimes sat down at her kitchen table; she created community, like the midwives on the Continent did, with the women and children who gathered inside and outside their huts while I interviewed them. When I told Shamburger about taking an hour and a half to get to her house when her directions said it would take 30 minutes, she told me, "I would have sent my brother-in-law to pick you up, but doing the kind of work you do, I thought you had to be white. I knew no white woman was going to get in the car with my brother-in-law." I smiled, remembering how several midwives I'd interviewed in Alabama expressed their pride in meeting a woman who had the support needed to move from New Jersey to Alabama for six months to interview Black midwives who were no longer in practice. At the time, Black women were just beginning to be seen on television as local reporters and news hosts.

When I returned to Alabama in 2019, I smiled, thinking how proud this midwife would be to know that a recorded interview with her sister, Annie Shamburger, RN, is on deposit at the Library of Congress (see Sonkin and Shambuger, *Annie Shamburger, Project Nurse, Talking about Health*). In the interview, she describes her public health work with the Farm Security Administration Federal Government Resettlement Project. The public health campaign included installing the first screens in cabins and providing families chickens and cows to address hunger and prevent sickness. Women living in crowded one-room cabins with multiple children were told to focus on ending the traditional kneeling birthing position that included stooping on pallets as their ancestors may have done on the Continent.

A lineage midwife, Shamburger also described how her mother, Rebecca Harriet Shamburger, who had moved to Africatown from Dallas County, introduced her to the extended responsibilities of midwifery care at an early age.

> SHAMBURGER: *My sister Annie Shamburger was a registered nurse, and she was the first Black registered nurse in Mobile County. And she worked there for about three years, and then she got on with the government Farm Program in Wilcox County. And then she sent for me to come up and help her. During that time, those folks was isolated in a section of Wilcox called Gees Bend. And when I was up there working with her, one of the famous doctors in Wilcox, a white doctor, asked me to go out and help deliver. So in the meantime, when I went out the first time I went out to deliver, I delivered twins, and that's how I began to start midwifery. I stayed up there nearly two years, and I came home. See, my mother was a midwife here in Mobile County, and she had been a midwife for about 40 years before I started.*
>
> *After I came home and I told her how many deliveries I had been with in Wilcox County, one of the doctors gave me a permit to go out with my mother. See, I had been going out with my mother before I left. I was interested in midwifery, but I was young, though, but I just went on out with her. I was not particular about becoming a midwife. See, I was sewing a lot. But as she practically had everything around here in the county, and sometimes she would go out and deliver, and my sister and I, we had to go back and bathe the babies, because she kept so busy.*

While in Mobile in 1981, I also met Louvenia Alberta Parker Taylor Benjamin, a midwife who lived in Loxley across the

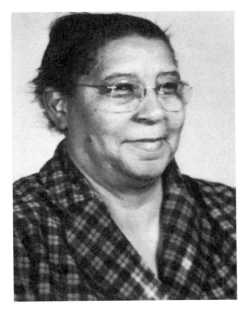

FIGURE 10.1. Louvenia Alberta Parker Taylor Benjamin's care for her patients shines through in this image.

bridge from downtown Mobile (see figure 10.1). Born in 1895, Benjamin attended the renowned Mobile Training High School in Africatown (just like Shamburger). After a day of teaching, Benjamin, a retired teacher and principal, remembered checking on newborn babies and mothers in the days immediately following a birth. Benjamin's postpartum care sometimes continued for weeks.

In the Jim Crow South, Benjamin advocated for mothers and confronted white doctors who denied that they needed medical attention. Years later, in Ethiopia, I would discover midwives who advocated for mothers and challenged hospital rules that deprived women of choosing a midwife for care or that failed to provide spaces for honoring traditions. In Loxley, 40 years earlier, Benjamin was confronting medical practices that reflected attitudes of white supremacy.

BENJAMIN: *So I asked Dr. Johnson because when I went there, Dr. Jordan wasn't there to look these babies over and see what you think about them. I said, "They were very small. Don't you think I should put them in the hospital or something?"*

"I'm not going to look at anything," he said. "I'm not a pediatrician. Take them to Mobile."

I said, "Where are these people going to get money to go to Mobile? They don't have any money to go to Mobile. They don't have any money to give me. I don't know any pediatricians in Mobile. All the doctors I know is here. You being a doctor, you could look at them."

When he said "No, I'm not going to touch them—I am not going to do anything," I said, "Well, I don't give a damn if you don't. I'll take them home and take care of them myself."

And I took those babies home and built a little nest for them. I put one in one end of the crib and one in the other. With some cloth and cotton, I built a nest for them. And there was an old lady that lived right next door to the child, and I asked her if she would take care of those babies while I was teaching, see, and I'd go every day to see about them.

I told her how to feed them. And I said, "And don't bother them until I come, and only change them if they need to be changed."

And you know, those babies are the finest things in the world. They're both grown now. And they're just fine, that boy and a girl. And I took care of those babies. I'd go by on my way out to the school. I'd go by and check in the mornings, and I'd come back in the afternoon and give them their baths. I didn't do much bathing to them, but I oiled them. And you know, they're the finest children, both of them. They're grown now and they're fine, fine children.

Benjamin also recalled managing other complicated births:

Now, I delivered triplets at Loxley. When I saw that third baby coming—I had delivered twins, but I hadn't delivered any triplets. And we tried and tried and tried and tried to get a doctor out there. I sent all around, "Tell the doctor to come here because I d[on't] know what to do," and I couldn't get a doctor. And when the doctor came, I had delivered all three of them, even dressed them, and they were identical. I couldn't tell one from the other, and they weighed the same amount of pounds. They all weighed seven pounds, and they are living now. They are men, and you can't hardly tell them apart now.

Willie Gray Taylor, now in her 70s, remembered leaving her job in Montgomery and coming home to Loxley so that her grandmother could deliver her baby in the house where she grew up. "I told my doctor, I had to go home because I wanted my grandmother to deliver the baby, so he sent the records to a doctor in Loxley and both doctors approved the idea," Taylor said. Once returning home, Taylor was reminded of the extent to which her grandmother was called on as a respected midwife in her community.

TAYLOR: *Day and night, folks would be coming to the house saying "I need Miss Beenie" [the nickname many in the community gave to Taylor's grandmother]. Screaming "I need Miss Beenie because so and so is having a baby now and she needs to come." I just thought she was just gracious teaching all day and anytime day or night she had to go and deliver a baby. My grandmother lived down the street from me. And she would just go all over, all over the county. A lot of them she taught, and she taught their parents. She would travel all over the place. They mostly paid her with goods. She wasn't working for the money. She shared a lot. She's the kind of person I want to be.*

About the unpredictability of knowing when a mother might begin labor, Benjamin said, "I told them when I took the job, when a mother needed me, that I would have to have someone else to cover my class."

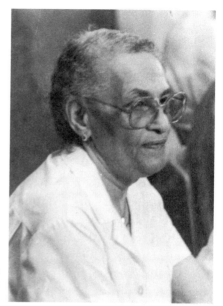

FIGURE 10.2. Julia Smith.
Photo used with permission
of © Debra Willis.

As a midwife and teacher, Benjamin was uniquely positioned to know children who became her future students. And mothers she waited on were previously students in the classes she taught. I learned from midwives on the Continent how the grandmother who assisted their mother at birth might also be the respected elder who chanted invocations and recited traditional poems. The voice of the respected elder was the midwife, the first voice the newborn heard.

Julia Smith, who worked as a midwife and domestic worker in Evergreen, Alabama, also vowed an unconditional commitment to her midwifery practice in ways that are similar to responding to a sacred calling (see figure 10.2). Smith prioritized responding to calls for birthing care over keeping her daytime job.

> SMITH: *I told the woman I was working for that if I had to go, I had to go and I would have to stay. If that wasn't acceptable, I didn't want the job. Now, I've private-home-worked lots. I was in the country; I worked in the field.*

After I come up here, I home-worked. Every time I took a job, any time they come and call, you got to be prepared. I got to go. I was working for one woman and she tried to yak-yak one day. Woman came right up in the middle of the day who needed a midwife, and she started yak-yak, and I said, "I told you this before. I told you I didn't want to work unless, when I get ready to go, I can go." I said, "I'm gone," and I left.

She didn't say nothing when I got back. Sometimes the labor is slow. That's one thing you can't urge. Now, I've always worked by myself. The thing that makes you say yes to it is something that the Lord put in the world, and somebody has got to take care of it. You don't know what kind of condition you're going into. If they want a midwife, it must be a person that is not able.

Growing up in Africatown, Darron Patterson remembered how Shamburger—who he always knew as "Mama Thelma"—not only served the community as a respected midwife but was also committed to meeting a range of needs as the "community doctor." Patterson's great-great-grandfather, Pollee Allen, was born in Africa and was one of the original inhabitants of Africatown. Patterson, president of the Clotilda Descendants Association, described Shamburger's courage and determination that contributed to her legacy as a midwife in Africatown.

PATTERSON: *I was born in Plateau, Alabama, and I was delivered by a midwife by the name of Miss Thelma Shamburger, "Mama Thelma." And she was the town doctor. Everybody went to her for everything medical. And she was just like everybody's mama, literally. Mama Thelma delivered just about everybody I know in Plateau.*

I thought Mama Thelma was a doctor. She even carried a black bag. We had other doctors like Dr. King on Highway 25, but in Plateau, if you needed something immediate, you went to Mama Thelma. She had home remedies.

*St. Martin de Porres—we called it Blessed Martin—that's
where some of the Black people used to go in Mobile, but
in Plateau for anything medical in Plateau, everyone went
to Mama Thelma. We respected her. She was the first face
a baby saw.*

Proteon Samuels, Shamburger's niece, had similar memories. "Mama Thelma had a remedy for everything," Samuels
explained. "And she had medical books. I remember when one
of the boys in the neighborhood cracked open his head on the
sidewalk. Everyone said, 'Go get Mama Thelma.' Back then,
you couldn't just walk up into some doctor's office." Samuels
remembered when white doctors seldom went to a Black woman's home to deliver her baby.

Patterson also described how Shamburger's life-long ties
with Dr. James A. Franklin, a leading Black physician, busi-
nessman, and civil rights activist, contributed to her community status. "He taught her well," Patterson said. "Dr. Franklin
was probably the premier Black doctor here. Dr. Franklin was
the man."

A 1954 edition of *Ebony* magazine features Dr. Franklin as
the "richest Negro doctor in the South." The article describes
how in the Jim Crow era, a parade of renowned activists, musicians, and famous athletes were welcomed to stay at the Franklin home. According to *Ebony,* Franklin's house guests included
Jackie Robinson, Marian Anderson, and Paul Robeson.

Pulling his cell phone out of his pocket as we talked, Patterson called Karlos Finley, attorney and part-time Mobile municipal judge, as well as Dr. Franklin's grandson, to arrange for a
meeting. Finley also heads the Dora Franklin Finley African
American Heritage Trail of Mobile, which includes a tour of
Africatown.

Meeting in the municipal judge's law office later that afternoon, Finley explained that his grandfather learned that a group
of white men in Evergreen, Alabama, were making plans to kill
him for touching a white woman. In 1917 Finley's grandfather

provided emergency medical care for a white woman because her husband could not afford to pay for a white doctor's medical care. Hoping to save Dr. Franklin's life, the patient's husband warned Dr. Franklin of threats to kill him and purchased a one-way train ticket for Dr. Franklin to travel as far away from Evergreen as possible. Dr. Franklin was accompanied by his wife and Finley's oldest uncle when making the harrowing escape.

> FINLEY: *Shamburger, who was only seven years old, spotted my grandfather walking down the dirt road from the Plateau train station and told him [Dr. Franklin], "I'm taking you home to Papa."*
>
> *So they lived with the Shamburger family until my grandfather was able to buy a doctor's office, which is where they lived.*
>
> *The only thing of value my grandfather had was a pocket watch which was given to him by his uncle when he got to Plateau [Africatown]. He sold that watch to purchase a blind mule and a wagon to do house calls.*

In a conversation filled with intimate "Mama Thelma" memories, Finley also described "Mama Thelma" as a community pillar.

> FINLEY: *Mama Thelma was a lifetime advocate for the health and well-being of her community. I witnessed it for myself. I've seen Mobile mayors call her the Mayor of Plateau; she was always a community leader. That goes back years, even before I was born.*

Shamburger's advocacy and community activism continued for decades after the state of Alabama decided to no longer issue midwife permits.

> FINLEY: *Whenever a political figure came to Plateau, they knew they needed to be ushered in by Mama Thelma. If*

they wanted their programs to be implemented, they had to talk to her first. She was a natural leader.

Even though I met Finley in 2019, more than 30 years after Shamburger's death, I felt like I could have been attending Shamburger's wake in Finley's office that afternoon—the lively kind of wake where stories evoking laughter and respect bring a person back to life.

When meeting with Shamburger's niece, later that evening, Samuels also reflected on her aunt's commitment to community and her spunk.

SAMUELS: *If you needed to get out of jail, get Social Security, hire a bailsman, get someone to get your birth certificate, you came to see Mama Thelma. And Mama Thelma got all the kids vaccinated. Mama Thelma brought all the kids to get vaccinated at the St. Matthew AME [African Methodist Episcopal] Church. Mama Thelma built that church right across from her house. It became the family church because there was no AME church in Africatown.*

So Miss Nellie Henderson, she was a nurse at the Board of Health, and Mama Thelma had the shots [vaccinations to be distributed] come here to the church. Then, when they started the Free Lunch Program, Mama Thelma had it at the church so all the children could get the free lunch for the first time. The church is not standing, but the cross stands up. We have had some bad hurricanes, but the cross never blew down.

As a midwife, Shamburger also made her home a birthing place for mothers who did not want to keep their babies.

SHAMBURGER: *I've delivered quite a few young girls right here, and they give the babies away and then go on back to school. Coming in from Montgomery and different places. Oh yes, plenty of them. Mm-hmm. And some of them I even take care of their babies and then give them away. I adopted one of them.*

Similar to women on the Continent, women in Africatown followed the ways of their ancestors in seeing the birth event as a time when women cared for women. On the Continent, midwives advocated for mothers who resented being forced to accept male doctors, nurses, or midwives as their caregivers when having to go to a facility or hospital to have their babies. Shamburger smiled recalling how her mother, a midwife, would never consent to a male caring for her as a birth attendant. In fact, her mother even left instructions about preparations for her burial that were gender specific, Shamburger (who also worked at funeral homes in the community making shawls for burials and as an embalmer) explained.

> SHAMBURGER: *She died right over there in the back room, and was embalmed in the back room and laid out the second day. See, I worked at the undertaker parlor too. Yeah, I've done quite a lot of embalming, helping cousin[s] out, then dress[ing] them. And she didn't want to go to the undertaker parlor because she said out of all 11 of her babies, no doctor never looked up her dress, and no man was going to touch her now.*

Like the midwives I met in Africa, Shamburger could not confirm the number of babies she or her mother had attended. About her 41 years as a midwife, Shamburger said, "now, they estimated when they had it in the paper here about two years ago, they counted up three thousand and something, but I don't know exactly." Recalling with laughter her busiest day as a midwife, Shamburger proudly described running from house to house.

> SHAMBURGER: *I have delivered as high as five babies a day, just jumping from house to house. Sure did. They all are all*

right, and they all are living. Now, Cleo was right back here on the next street, and Mary was over there on Lincoln Avenue. And when the pastor found out I was over here with Cleo, I had just finished with Cleo, then went on over to Mary Love, finished with Mary Love and went back down through the pecan orchard. Then from the pecan orchard, I went over to deliver twins.

Shamburger, president of the Mobile Midwife Club for 30 years, died on August 28, 1998. Shamburger's niece remembered listening to testimonials from community members who came into the world guided by Shamburger's hands. "When the pastor asked for everyone who was delivered by Shamburger to stand, the whole church stood up," Samuels said. In the early 1980s, Shamburger had participated in a historic meeting supported by the United Methodist Church at the Women's Resource Center at Spelman College, a Historically Black College, that honored Shamburger as well as Margaret Charles Smith from Eutaw, Julia Smith from Evergreen, and other Black midwives I met in Alabama who collectively had attended thousands of births in their communities. At the first independent meeting of former Black midwives in Alabama, Black feminist and scholar Beverly Guy-Sheftall, Deborah Willis (an internationally renowned Black photographer and now chair of the Department of Photography at New York University), and I collaborated in planting seeds for ongoing projects to document the significance of historically Black midwifery practices. Willis was also eager to join the Spelman meeting because her grandmother, Lilian Foreman Holman, had delivered babies in the Philadelphia community where she lived.

When the Spelman meeting was held, I did not know that Louvenia Taylor Benjamin, the respected teacher, principal, and midwife, was no longer alive. Over coffee with Willie Gray Taylor at Burger King, I learned that her grandmother, Benjamin, had died on September 1, 1981, just ten days after I interviewed her, at the age of 86. Though she had used a cane, she walked with a straight back in a way that demanded respect. Although unable to find the key to open her desk drawer where she kept the article that she had clipped from the local newspaper about her decades of midwifery practice, Benjamin said that the paper reported her delivering more than a thousand babies.

Recalling how mothers continued to seek her services long after the state of Alabama made it illegal for lay midwives to practice, Benjamin said, "I've had about eight white people come here since they cut me off. They wanted me to deliver. All those that I have delivered, they want me again." With water barely visible at the edges of her eyes, Benjamin spoke with pride, not sadness. "My last two I delivered was in Fairhope, white babies," Benjamin said. "They bring them to see me every birthday."

Our meeting ended with the former director of the Macedonia Baptist Church Choir singing softly: "I'm happy with Jesus alone. Though poor and deserted, thank God I can say, I'm happy with Jesus alone." Surely Benjamin's hums comforted countless mothers in labor and her prayers were powerful spiritual towers that mothers leaned on.

BENJAMIN: *I'd just say, "Lord, now you come here, 'cause I can't do this by myself." I'd just talk to him like I was talking to another man. And I don't care when any of them would come and tell me that they were in labor, I'd get on my knees and tell the Lord about it.*

I'd say, "Now Lord I got to go out to get this baby." I say, "I can't get him by myself. You have to help me." And they usually come out all right. O yeah, I prayed. I pray yet. I pray, pray almost constantly, 'cause I'm here by myself, and I just pray to the Lord, take care of me, and you know, nobody bothers me.

Well, the 23rd Psalm is my favorite scripture, and sometimes I quote the first psalm that I know by heart. They're my favorite scriptures. The Lord is my shepherd, and I always say I don't have to want.

As far back as we have written and oral records, priest-
esses, midwives, and esteemed elders who assisted at birth
transformed themselves into instruments calling on spiritual
forces for protection and purification of the birthing space.
Midwives on the Continent poured libations, chanted invocations, and called on their deities and the Creator with names
preserved in their precolonial languages. When I visited Jennifer Houser Wegner, associate curator in the Egyptian Section
at the University of Pennsylvania Museum of Archaeology and
Anthropology, she described a wand in their collection that
was used to evoke protection from goddesses and deities more
than 5,000 years earlier (see figure 10.3). As I held the ancient
Egyptian Magical Birth Wand in my gloved hands, images of
the hippopotamus, "the great one of the Nile," and lotus flow-
ers—symbols of purity, enlightenment, and regeneration of
body mind and spirit and the daily rebirth of the sun—briefly
created a space of purity and enlightenment in a museum lab
in Philadelphia. Wegner also explained that in ancient Egypt,
wands and clappers adorned with symbols of birth and regeneration were sometimes buried with the dead. As I listened to
her explain the Egyptian wand symbols, in my mind I heard
my grandmother speaking to me decades ago, before her death,
as she sat on her porch. When Wegner spoke about the wand
as a magical instrument, I saw lotuses flying in the air, a hippopotamus crossing the Nile, and other images she described
rising off the wand just like, in the same way, I had once seen
my ancestors riding in a carriage beyond a fence as my grandmother described them.

WEGNER: *The wand is decorated with a whole set of protective images including various deities or semidivine char-
acters. Probably the one that is most identifiable looks like
a hippopotamus. There's a goddess by the name of Tawaret,
whose name means the "Great Female One," who is symbolized by the hippopotamus here. There are also images of
the desert cat and vultures, which is the hieroglyphic word*

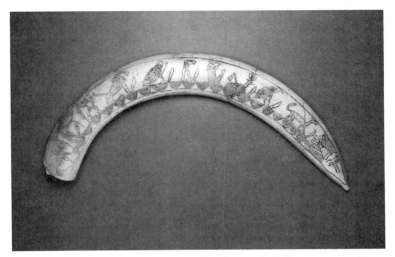

FIGURE 10.3. Ancient Egyptian Magical Birth Wand of Hippopotamus Ivory, from Rifeh, Egypt, dating to the Middle Kingdom (ca. 1991–1778 BCE). Image courtesy of the University of Pennsylvania Museum of Archaeology and Anthropology, Accession Number E2914.

used for "mother." And there is an image of a frog representing the goddess Heqet. It is thought that these wands were used during the birthing process and that a practitioner would draw a circle in the sand around the place where the woman is laboring and that that encircled space would be sort of magically protecting her. And all of these gods and goddesses on here would also help with that protection . . . This might be a lotus flower. The Egyptians did a lot with the lotus. It was an important symbol of rebirth and regeneration.

✳

Before traveling to Africa in 2019, I met with Chester Higgins Jr., a *New York Times* photographer for more than four decades whose books provided positive images focusing on the life and culture of people of African descent. As I sat talking with him

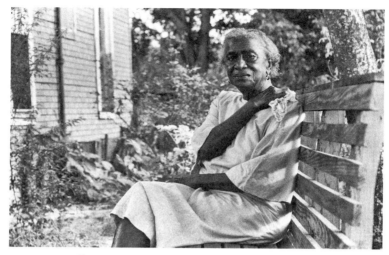

FIGURE 10.4. Chester Higgins captures the spirit of Aunt Shugg Lampley. Image used with permission of © Chester Higgins. Courtesy of the Bruce Silverstein Gallery.

and his wife, Betsy Kissam, in their Brooklyn brownstone, surrounded by large elephant leaf plants, Chester recalled his reverence for the wisdom of Black elders he knew when he was growing up. The renowned photographer also showed me books in his collection that described birthing and medicinal practices of ancient Egyptians. Our conversation influenced the work I later did in Africa. As we talked, Higgins explained that when he photographs, his challenge is to reveal the presence of the spirit.

In Higgins's photography book *Echo of the Spirit*, Shugg Lampley, an Alabama midwife, is depicted kneeling in prayer, which is how many midwives prepared themselves to call on the Spirit within the birthing space. In this image, Higgins, a photographer known for images that portray the resilience, spirit, and dignity of people of African American and African descent, captures the spirit of "Aunt Shugg," who was like a mother to him (see figure 10.4). "Aunt Shugg was associated with everything sweet like the blueberries she picked to make blueberry pie and the peppermint candy she kept in her pockets to give children whenever she was standing by her front yard gate," Higgins told me when I spoke with him in 2019 about his grandmother. Higgins recalled that "Aunt Shugg" was not only called on to support mothers and babies in the birth room but that she was called on when someone in the family or community was approaching death. "Aunt Shugg and her brother, Uncle March Fourth McGowan, could predict by the signs of the moon when it was time for them to 'sit' with the sick," Higgins said. "Anyone could take the day shift, but Aunt Shugg and Uncle Fourth took the night shift so a person would have a 'good death,' as people called it."

Higgins continued, "When Aunt Shugg walked into the church sanctuary, everyone stood up out of respect." Bowing his head, he added, "I also remember how people saluted her with a bow whenever they passed her house."

Just like I met with Higgins before I traveled to the Continent in 2019, I met with Sarah Penn before traveling to Alabama in 1981. Like Higgins, Penn was a longtime New Yorker who also revered her ancestral family midwife. Penn was the owner of Knobkerry, a trend-setting shop that opened in the Lower East Side in the early 1960s. On the Saturday morning that I dropped in, Sarah's shop, a popular gathering place and salon for Black poets, artists, and unorthodox musicians, including Ornette Coleman, had not yet filled with customers as she told me how congressmen and others had recognized the contributions of her midwife grandmother Sadie Lee.

In 1974 in Childersburg, Alabama, hundreds gathered for the dedication ceremony of the Sadie Lee Homes and Community Center in honor of Sadie Lee, a midwife, teacher, and community pillar. The Sadie Lee Homes and Community Center became the first integrated center in Childersburg. Anne Penn, Lee's daughter, told a newspaper reporter, "There was only one doctor in this little community then, about 3,000 people." Penn recalled, "Mother went down to Tuskegee Institute and studied the profession of midwifery to help the doctor. After a while the doctor would just say 'Call Sadie,' when the time came." She continued, "The county records showed she had delivered more than 2,000 babies, both white and Black." Lee delivered her last baby at the age of 90.

As a midwife committed to community advocacy, Lee opened a school on the second floor of her house, where she taught farmers how to manage their farms, sell their products, and read and write. In the spirit of self-help touted by Booker T. Washington, Lee later joined with her daughter in opening a community center that included classes on piano, sewing, canning, home economics, landscaping, and crafts. On Sundays, the center was used for Sunday school classes and vesper worship. Lee's daughter said, "Mother believed in education and did all she could to inspire her family and all other young people to get an education." Lee raised a total of twenty-one children; six of them were adopted.

Midwives on the Continent and across the diaspora whose wisdom and holistic practices extended beyond birthing are ubiquitous.

Toni Morrison, a midwife descendant, described the authority of her great-grandmother, a midwife, in a 1983 conversation with Nellie McKay published in *Conversations with Toni Morrison*. The novelist and essayist remembered how her great-grandmother—who had no formal education—was respected for her medical knowledge:

> I remember that when my grandmother walked into a room, her grandsons and her nephews stood up. The women in her family were very, very articulate. Of course, my great-grandmother could not read, but she was a midwife, and people from all over the state came for her advice and for her to deliver babies. They came for other kinds of medical care too. Yes, I feel the authority of those women more than I do my own.

Africatown's story of resilience was hidden from world view for more than a century, as were the birthing traditions and ceremonies of the town's ancestors born in West Africa. On the Continent, midwives described the practice of bowing and kneeling out of respect for midwives whenever they passed them on the road. The stories that Higgins, Penn, and Morrison shared spotlight how ancestral midwives in their families won respect and honor in the Black communities they served.

CHAPTER 11

Hampton to Charlottesville

Rebirthing Midwife Traditions

Just as the COVID restrictions of 2021 began to lift, I updated my pre-pandemic plans to interview midwife descendants and doulas who are continuing some traditional midwife practices in Virginia. Living in Hampton, Virginia, I frequently walk at Fort Monroe. I still feel the presence of the spirits of the first enslaved Africans who landed there. Fort Monroe was declared Freedom's Fortress near the end of the Civil War. Enslaved pregnant Black mothers walked miles to reach Fort Monroe; they knew that if their babies were born in the largest contraband camp in the US on the Chesapeake Bay's banks at Freedom's Fortress, their child would be born free.

Some of the earliest colonial plantation records documenting midwife practices are found in Virginia. While there were many more births within the enslaved community than there are entries in Thomas Jefferson's *Farm Book,* Jefferson records paying a midwife, Rachael, $2.00 for births she attended on the Monticello plantation in Charlottesville. Believed to have been born on the Shadwell property owned by Jefferson's parents, Rachael played a significant role as a midwife at Monticello between 1813 and 1825. For example, in 1825 Rachael was paid for being a midwife to "Anne, the daughter of Wormley and

Ursula and also caring for Maria," who Jefferson notes was "the daughter of Joe Fosset and Edy." Both of these enslaved families made significant contributions to Jefferson, which included performing skillful work on the plantation and supporting Jefferson at the White House.

I went to Charlottesville, Virginia, in the spring of 2021 to interview midwife descendants and mothers who'd received care from traditional midwives when giving birth in the 1940s and '50s.

Although there are no Black midwives practicing in Charlottesville now, there are initiatives to continue traditions that are at the heart of historic midwifery practices. Doulas, for example, also aim to develop relationships with the women they serve that promote trust, respect, and communication throughout their pregnancy and birthing experience.

When visiting Charlottesville in 2019, I noticed an abundance of signs pointing to vineyards, apple orchards, and mountain climbing. By 2021 the road into Charlottesville was a highway marked by countless Black Lives Matter signs and flags, a powerful reminder that this time of racial reckoning is also the time for the stories of Black midwives in Virginia to come into the light of day.

I met Flora Ragland Washington, 85 years old, the first midwife descendant I interviewed in Cobham, Louisa County, a 30-minute drive from downtown Charlottesville. Surprised to find the church locked, Washington suggested that we sit in her car, Betsy, to talk. With the car radio tuned to a station playing gospel music, Washington described the community where she grew up and how her family's ties to the community extended back to the era of enslavement. Licensed as a midwife in 1933, her mother, Earline Elliott Lewis Ragland Maupin, served mothers whose families sometimes had existing bonds with her family, which fostered trust, respect, and communication. Although Maupin's family was well known and respected in the community prior to her becoming a midwife, respect for Maupin grew as she provided leadership in a community effort to provide bus services for young children, including those she'd delivered.

> WASHINGTON: *So we're in Louisa County, but up on the upper edge of Louisa County, where we're almost close to Albemarle County, a skip, hop, and jump. I grew up in this area right here, born and raised. We lived here until my grandfather passed. My mother lived in the old home place right down here behind us. You can see where I was born and raised at. We have an old church down there. I think they started building on this church here in the 1960s. All this through here my grandfather owned. The other house too, down below the other house on the other side, all this he owned. And the church was built down on his property for years. When white people burned up the House of God Church that Black people went to, that's when my father became Pentecostal. Back years ago, he heard God's calling . . .*
>
> *Oh yes, oh yes. My family—my mother and grandfather—it was well known [that] if somebody got sick, they would sit with them in the home and do for them. My grandfather was a good friend and that type of stuff. People would call him for sickness in the family. If somebody was sick and they wasn't getting well, they would call on him to come for prayer. He grabbed that old black robe. You'd see Grandpa walking, going to somebody's house for prayer day and night for him come for prayer. He kept faithful. People would call him for sickness in the family and they would get well. Sometimes my brother and I would walk with him. My grandfather couldn't read. He kept his faith in God . . .*
>
> *My grandmother, I think she did some midwifing along with a sister she had. Somebody named Lena. My grandmother was a Mahane. And she still has a lot of kin people through this area. Her mother was a Black lady, and her father was white . . .*

I think my mother might [have] had a third-grade education. Back then that was doing something. I know she could read and write, but I don't know how much education she had because if you had a third-grade education you had something. When I started school, they had a school bus for white children, but Black children always had to walk. It was a long way and it was hard. My mother went to meetings to raise money for a school bus, so we didn't have to walk to school . . .

I don't have any of the record books from her being a midwife. I do have some pictures of her down in Louisa—'cause that's where she'd go to have meetings and things. I do have those. And I know there's a lotta Black ladies in that picture with her. But I do not know any names because at that time I'm young, and I know my momma be gone could be a couple days or maybe a day or she may be gone one night.

But she was blessed. I think she only lost one child during her being a midwife—and that's because she had called the doctor. The doctor came in, and he wouldn't listen to her. So the baby passed. I think the girl passed too or whatever. She said I kept telling him that this lady needed to go to the hospital, and he wouldn't listen. He kept saying, "No, no, no, no." I do know she always talked about that.

Yeah. They learned. Not only on people, but they learned on animals. I remember when I was much younger, we had a cow who couldn't have the calf. At that time, I was about 14 or 15. My granddaddy came to the house. Never called her Erlene. Her nickname was Bunky. He called her. Said, "I need you." She went down there. Next thing you hear that little calf hollering. The cow couldn't have the calf. Momma delivered the calf. She was able to save that calf and the cow, and that type of stuff. She only lost that one, and that wasn't her fault.

It's impossible to know how many babies she delivered. I'm trying to think. Oh, we often thought about that as we

*got older. If they had just kept a record of how many babies
my momma brought in. But I think really my momma
brought into the world just about every child around here
in this section.*

Before returning to my car, Washington suggested that we
walk back to the old family home place near the original church
that her grandfather built. Some of the mothers she delivered,
like Maxine Holland's mother, would visit or attended Maupin's church. Holland said, "She delivered just about everybody
around here including me." In a 2018 Juneteenth ceremony, the
Cobham community recognized Maupin's longtime service as
a midwife.

✳

Born enslaved on the Page plantation near Cobham in 1835,
Elizabeth Carter died at 102 in 1933, the same year Maupin
began her midwife practice. Gloria Gilmore, Louisa County
historian and a midwife descendant herself, explained that
Carter is still remembered in her community as the midwife
"who lived on top of the mountain." Much of the land she once
owned remains in the Carter family, and Gilmore explained
that the road where Carter's house was located was named
Carter Winkey Lane. Carter and many of her family members
are buried in the Carter family cemetery on Carter's former
property. In an article announcing her death published in the
Orange Review, a local white-owned weekly newspaper, Carter
is described as "serving as a slave until freedom was declared
before living at various places in Louisa, Albemarle and Orange
Counties."

   L. Teresa Church, Ph.D., a poet, independent archivist, and
playwright, described how her family's long-standing relationships with families in Hubbards Hill, Virginia, also extended
back to the era of enslavement. Her grandmother, Mary Simuel
Martin Morse, who was born in 1879, cared for mothers whose

ancestors worked as sharecroppers and were once enslaved on the same plantation as her family's ancestors.

> CHURCH: *My grandmother, Mary Simuel Martin Morse, lived on the property that was once part of a large plantation. It was parceled up and sold to members of her family and others. My paternal grandfather, Thomas Henry Morse, helped to lead the community campaign to build the first Little Zion Baptist Church on property that he purchased from the Hubbard family. Later, the first school to serve the Black community was built across the road from the church.*
>
> *My grandmother's mother was born enslaved, and my grandmother delivered mothers whose parents also were enslaved on the same plantation, so the families knew one another. When their grandparents died, the family would bury them in the old slave burial ground adjoining the property that was once part of the plantation.*
>
> *Grandma [Morse] would sometimes prepare a repast at the old house that goes back to where my grandparents used to live. People from my grandparents' generation would walk back to the old house for whatever my grandmother would fix. Grandma would have on a clean dress and a clean apron, and she might have prepared biscuits or hoe cakes and put out preserves, pickles, and jelly in those little dishes to help make a biscuit taste good.*

Church was the only midwife descendant I interviewed in Virginia who came into the world through the hands of her grandmother, just like several of the traditional midwives I interviewed on the Continent.

> CHURCH: *My grandmother delivered me. I was the last baby born in the house where my father was born. My father's truck was not in good enough shape to drive down the highway to Charlottesville to get to the hospital, so he*

decided to go across the river to get his brother to take Mother to the hospital. By the time he returned 30 minutes later, I was born. They said I was the baby who was born in a hurry. They said I was put in the bed hollering, welcoming myself—announcing my presence in the world. I was the last baby she delivered.

Respect for the midwife also stemmed from long-standing informal relationships even when there were no family ties. Some mothers established relationships with the midwife, which came from being a longtime neighbor. When Louise Rush was born in Howardsville, 26 miles south of Charlottesville, the midwife who delivered her was someone who had an established informal relationship with her family. In a 2002 interview that was part of the University of Virginia Race and Place Project, Rush remembered Roberta Barrett as the midwife who "brought us here." Rush explained, "She lived in a little house, but you couldn't see it because of the trees, but we wasn't too far apart . . . Everybody who was born . . . she brought us here." When Rush later went to Esmont, Jessie Coleman was the midwife she knew and trusted when she had her babies at home.

> RUSH: *Well, I had all of them here—all of them except for the last two. Those were my last ones: Patrick and Pearl, the twins. The twins, yeah. And I probably would have had them here, but my midwife, she had done passed on. She was deceased when they were born . . . Mm-hmm, them were the only two. The rest I had at home.*

M. Waltine Eubanks, in an interview in Charlottesville, also recalled the respect women had for Coleman as a midwife, a person who was confident in her skills and did not bow down to the white doctors and nurses in the community. Eubanks added that women she knew were often disappointed with the care they received at the University of Virginia Hospital.

EUBANKS: *She [Jessie Coleman] was blessed and highly favored, as the scripture says. She was sort of put on a pedestal because without Miss Jessie you didn't survive birthing your child. That's all you had. That's all you knew. She was most active in the Chestnut Grove Community because that's where she lived. She had a big, beautiful two-story house. In a way, she was sort of well-off. You would say that by today's standards. By those days' standards, if you could build a house with more than three rooms, you were considered well-off. I know she was paid, but it wasn't always money because a lot of times it was a country ham, some chicken, or some eggs.*

She birthed most of the babies in four different communities—Esmont, Chestnut Grove, Howardsville, and Scottsville. I finally knew her when I was about seven or eight. She was a very stately fair-skinned woman with beautiful crinkly hair . . . She was very intelligent, and see, she didn't take any mess. If you were going to waste her time, bye-bye.

She had to be tough. She was serious about her craft, and she was not going to be disrespected. It didn't matter whether you were the doctor or the nurse; you were going to respect her. She spoke up. She wasn't mealy-mouthed; she was not afraid to express her opinion, so for a Black person doing that in the 40s, you were thought to be crazy . . .

In my opinion I think the mother felt safer with somebody she knew or who knew the family. The mother knew she would receive the best treatment that was available. When in the hospital, it is just cold, sterile, and you are being told to "hurry up and plop that thing out, I got somebody else to go to."

Eubanks knew that when the University of Virginia Hospital opened in 1901, it was built to provide medical care for white patients only. In *Notes on the State of Virginia,* Thomas Jefferson, the founder of University of Virginia, touted pseudo biological and intellectual differences between whites and Blacks. These ideas fueled long-lasting ideologies that promoted justifying eugenics and segregation at the University of Virginia.

Systemic racism at UVA Hospital continued to limit employment opportunities for Blacks in the 20th century. For example, in the 1940s, Black women were restricted to jobs as ward maids under the supervision of white nurses and were paid $7.00 a week. The first Black nurse did not graduate from the UVA School of Nursing until 1970. In the 1950s Black women giving birth at UVA Hospital were restricted to a segregated ward in the hospital basement known as Ward Q.

Born in 1925, Teresa Jackson Walker Price (in her 90s when I interviewed her in 2021) chose to have her baby at the University of Virginia Hospital in 1951 (see figure 11.1). I met Price, a retired teacher and the first Black librarian hired to work in the desegregated Charlottesville school system, at her home in Charlottesville, a few blocks from Vinegar Hill, a neighborhood that once included Charlottesville's vibrant downtown business district but was leveled by urban renewal in the 1960s. Believing it was her right as a Black woman to give birth at the UVA Hospital, Price described how role models in her family instilled in her the resilience, pride, and determination needed to take a stand and seek care at a hospital with a long history of treating Blacks unfairly. When birthing with a community-based midwife, women often had previous bonds with midwives and their families. Although Price and her family had long-standing relationships with the few Black doctors in the community, those doctors could not obtain privileges at UVA Hospital because of their race. Price described her family's long history of contributing to the Black community in Charlottesville and how she tapped into her family history of resilience when deciding to give birth at UVA Hospital.

> PRICE: *My grandmother is a Charlottesville native. A school, Jackson Via Elementary School, is named for her because she was a recognized and respected teacher. The*

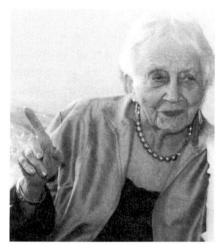

FIGURE 11.1. Teresa Jackson
Walker Price

school is named for two ladies who were teachers. My grandmother was a Black teacher and Ms. Via was a white teacher. When they put the name on the school, they chose a name from each part of the community and that kept everybody quiet . . .

So where you are sitting right now used to be a doctor's office. My father built this house as a duplex because there were no Black doctors here at the time, and he was determined to attract a Black doctor to come work in Charlottesville. He thought if they knew they had a space for setting up an office, that would encourage them to move to Charlottesville. So when I was growing up, there was always a doctor next door.

Our teachers in our schools supplied those things that they realized we didn't have access to. And I will always admire those teachers for that. If there were things that were going on—state competitions and so forth that were going on for white students—the Black teachers made it possible for their students to do the same thing . . . We need to remember the work that the midwives did. People always stepped up.

During Price's childbearing years, however, the UVA Hospital denied Black doctors hospital privileges, and women could either choose a midwife for home birthing care or be forced to have their babies in the segregated UVA Hospital basement's boiler room.

PRICE: *When I came along that was in 1951, you had a Black doctor in the city who made some connections for you at the hospital. Well, we had three [Black doctors]. And I was able to get a good obstetrician from the University of Virginia, a doctor who did take Black patients. So I got some prenatal care. And he delivered the child, I think. That doctor should have been there to deliver that baby, but it's a training hospital.*

When the delivery actually approached, you took yourself to the hospital . . . We were relegated to the basement. We had a ward, no private rooms. And sometimes it was crowded. And the pipes—the heating pipes were visible from your bedside. So that was not pleasant. Of course, at that time with what you were doing, you weren't paying much attention to a pipe.

No water ever dripped on me. But you always heard stories of how you had to duck the dripping water. I didn't experience that . . . But the actual delivery was upstairs in the sterile section . . .

One of the public health nurses here, Mrs. Imogene Bunn, whose husband was the minister at First Baptist Church, was very instrumental in opening up facilities for us to get better care. Rev. Benjamin Bunn was the pastor at First Baptist Church on Main Street. I say that because there's also a First Baptist Church that was white.

So they paved the way for us getting out of the basement.

While court cases and protests led to the end of Jim Crow segregation in health care facilities, inequities in treatment, high infant and maternal morbidity and mortality rates, and access to quality and wholistic health care remain a concern for Black women and other women of color in Charlottesville and the nation. The Birth Sisters of Charlottesville, a collective of women of color, aims to improve birthing outcomes for Black women by providing an array of ongoing physical, social, and psychological/spiritual supports grounded in relationships that reflect trust and mutual respect.

Just as midwife descendants described how midwives in their families tapped into prayer and other spiritual practices, doulas often recommend that mothers tap into mantras, meditation, and affirmations to reduce stress. Brown Baby Bump Love Baths, where a mother is advised to take time out to focus on sending love to her baby while the infant "is still growing in her belly," is one of the practices described by Doreen Bonnet, a doula and the Birth Sisters' executive director.

The community-based doula said that pregnant women who never practiced meditation or mindfulness techniques prior to their pregnancy appreciate a doula's guidance to take time out to wrap their baby in a blanket of love even before the baby is born.

Bonnet also explained how she sometimes taps into her reiki practice when supporting mothers during pregnancy, labor, and birth. Similar to traditional midwives on the Continent whose holistic practices were respected in the community, Bonnet explained how she comes from a Louisiana family of traiteurs (or treateurs), who are known for their laying on of hands and use of touch for healing.

> BONNET: *So, a couple of years ago the doula collective was offering free training for doulas. At the time when I saw the posting for it, I didn't know what a doula really was. I was giving the flyers to other people and I thought to*

check this out. Once I looked at it and found out what it was, I said that's naturally who I am. I said I'm naturally a healing person. I am someone who naturally wants to be present with people during a process like that. It is about my ability to be present. I let mothers know I'm right there with them. I let them know that I understand what they are going through. I tell them, "I'm with you. I'm going to get you through this."

Now doulas and midwives across the country are lobbying for state and national legislation that seeks to improve birth outcomes for women of color. Along with supporting mothers before, during, and for a short period after birth, this organization also defines addressing systemic racism that leads to inequities in health care outcomes as part of its mission.

Museums across the country are now recognizing the practices of traditional midwives. The stories of traditional midwives in Alabama and across the South document a long history of advocating for mothers when white doctors failed to treat their Black patients in dignified ways.

The Mobile Medical Museum, with its sculpture of midwife hands in Mobile, Alabama; the Lucy Jacobs Midwife Memorial in Liberty, Missouri; the Scott Ford House, telling the story of Virginia Ford, a midwife in Jackson, Mississippi; and the Smithsonian Museum of African American History and Culture that recognizes the contributions of enterprising and legendary midwife Mary Coley, of Albany, Georgia, and Claudine Curry Smith, a Virginia midwife, are examples of the growing recognition of historical African American midwifery practices. Simultaneously, increasing numbers of contemporary African American midwives are choosing to embrace some of the timeless birthing traditions sustained by midwives of African descent who preceded them.

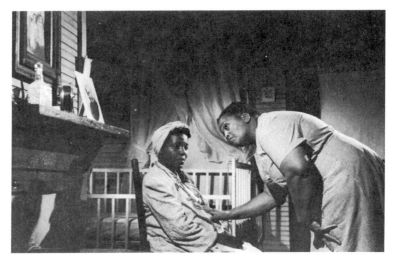

FIGURE 11.2. Miss Mary Coley times contractions in "Timing Contractions," a photograph from Robert Galbraith's *Reclaiming Midwives: Stills from "All My Babies."* Used by permission of Robert Galbraith.

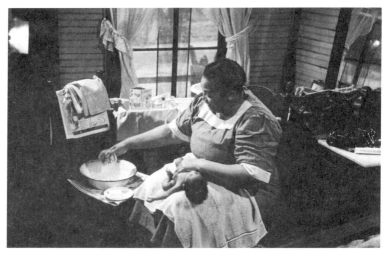

FIGURE 11.3. Miss Mary Coley bathes a newborn infant in "Next Day Continuing Care," a photograph from Robert Galbraith's *Reclaiming Midwives: Stills from "All My Babies."* Used by permission of Robert Galbraith.

Living in New York at the time of her children's birth, Panya Walker, Teresa Jackson Walker Price's granddaughter, told me why she gave birth at home with the support of a midwife and a doula because she did not trust her obstetrician to respect her birth plan.

> WALKER: *My doctor was focused on everything that could go wrong. She said I was overweight. She said I was having multiple births. She said I was high-risk. The doctor was seeing negativity every step of the way. The focus was on what the speculum could touch, ultrasound, coldness and wires and no laying on of hands or touch. I didn't feel safe in that context . . . my age, my weight, then I was having twins put me in a high-risk category. For me, going to the hospital didn't feel safe. Because I felt the threat of going under the knife. My obstetrician focused on the risks— twins usually present breech, the likelihood that you will have a C-section. It didn't feel like a potentiality. It felt like a probability . . . It felt like a bait-and-switch. I believe there was more than one [doctor] that I interviewed, and the message tended to be "we'll do our best, but you'll probably need a C-section." I felt pressured, so I began to explore different options . . . I chose to give birth at home, and the midwife assured me that we could get to a hospital quickly if there was a need. My midwife had also delivered many twins through home birth, and that was reassuring to me.*

Born in Hopewell, Virginia, Michelle Drew (see figure 11.4) is a nurse midwife with a long history of championing greater recognition of Black midwives and supports women choosing to give birth at home. Now practicing as a midwife in Delaware, much of what she learned from her grandmother's practice as a Virginia midwife is reflected in her ways of caring for and supporting women during pregnancy and birth. As co-chair of the American College of Nurse-Midwives Truth and Reconciliation Task Force, Drew recommends establishing midwifery training

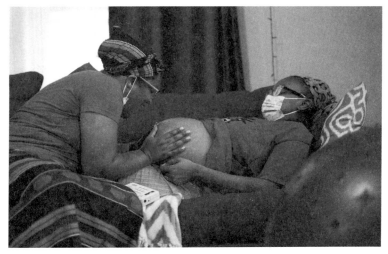

FIGURE 11.4. Midwife Michelle Drew with client Amber Twyne, receiving at-home prenatal care. Permission © Quantizing Kareem, photographer.

programs that recognize and incorporate some of the traditions and practices of historic traditional Black midwives into the curriculum at Historically Black Colleges and Universities.

> DREW: *I think as Black midwives we have to recognize that we need to be the nexus, we need to be the center of regrowing the midwifery workforce. The system that eliminated an entire workforce of more than 100,000 Black women in a very short period of time cannot be trusted to just be magnanimous and say, "Oh, you're right; we were wrong; we're sorry; here." So I think we need to put those powers, that origin, into Black institutions. I think we need midwifery programs at Historically Black Colleges and Universities. I'm an unapologetic proponent in saying that there need not be another nurse midwifery program accredited by the American College of Nurse-Midwives until there are at least two HBCUs. Because predominantly white institutions have already proven that their job is either to tolerate us or, in many situations, to keep us out . . .*

I remember walking around town with my grand-mother as a very small child. Of course, everyone greeted my granny. Everyone revered her. I remember people driv-ing and pulling up just to greet her.

In a town like Hopewell in the summertime, one of your primary activities is just sitting on the front porch watching the world go by. And having folks pull up and ask her advice on things, ask her opinions on things. It could have been about finance, it could've been what was happ[en]ing in the political situation. People respected her opinion . . . People revered her. A day seldom went by that somebody just wouldn't pull up and say, "I just came from fishing with a bag full of catfish." Or "We're bringing in our garden, and here's corn or beans."

So she also is the person that I knew who was really tied to the community—a servant to her community. In all different aspects, I knew her as a caregiver. I remem-ber even as a child growing up that what was probably the most important thing about her life was that she took care of the church. Whether it was being committed to the physical structure of the church or teaching the children in the church, she was a committed person to her community.

At Friendship Baptist Church on Arlington Road, she taught Sunday school, and of course she was a member of the usher board and was a senior usher. At some point she served as the president of the usher board. I remember when growing up that one of my goals in life was to be an usher. That posture and those white gloves. But it was like so much an extension of who she was. Even in leadership. She always had that air walking around—I've seen pictures of me lately, and I stand like her now. The habit I have of just walking around the community here and just walking through to see our neighbors and to know what's going on. I think I got a lot of that from her.

She knew the people to talk to, and she had that agency through her work and through her extension of really what was a ministry to her to make connections. We've lost that.

Yeah, the caring that she gave extended far beyond just taking care of you when you were pregnant or birthing, or even when they were treating the sick. Midwives were respected for their wisdom. By the time they became [a] midwife, they were seasoned and entered the practice as elders. So they held that position . . .

She prayed continuously. She had no compunction of praying out loud while she had her hands on people. She blessed babies. She anointed bellies. Her connection to her Creator was strong, and it was really central to her being. I'm sure a good number of people in her care and in our community were nominally—perhaps they weren't as tied to her faith and tradition as she was, but she didn't care. She prayed over you. And I've been known to do that too. That's another one of the things that I learned from her.

I have one vague memory. And sometimes I wonder if it's real or was it in my mind of, you know, going with her. Because I was the runt of the litter, of the grandchildren, I often had to go places with her. So I do have a memory of being in a place where I'm pretty sure it was a birth. Or maybe it was just a visit. I remember sitting in a corner and playing with this woman's children and seeing my grandmother. One of the first things that she did was put her hands on a mother. Laying on of hands and praying for a mother and baby.

Wrapped in the mystery of life and death is birth. She relied a lot on God and in her faith in God.

✳

Back in Hampton and just a couple of miles away from where I live, Chauncey Brown, lifetime Hampton resident and a midwife descendant, told me how Rosie Callis Brown, his great-grandmother, extended her care to women for decades.

I interviewed Brown at his home in Phoebus, overlooking the Chesapeake Bay where enslaved Africans arrived after a tortuous journey from Angola. Surely, some of the women or their descendants who arrived on the *White Lion* became midwives like Brown's great-grandmother.

BROWN: *My great-grandmother Rosa Callis Brown was a noted midwife in this area.*

Born in Matthews County, she and her husband were married in 1872, so she was not that far removed from the time of slavery and carried on the things that she was taught by her foreparents.

I talked with elders here who told me that my great-grandmother was an herbalist as well. So the plot of land that they bought is still wooded, and at this point, I still have that property.

I would imagine that she could go back out in the woods on the property where they lived and pick the herbs that she needed. The actual address is 916 Quash Street, and the extent of it runs from Quash Street all the way back to North King Street. There were a couple of other midwives that I knew of, but she was the one that serviced the Old North Hampton area, and that's the area surrounding Quash Street and King Street . . .

One of the things that seems to be unique, but it is probably more common that we know, and we have factual evidence of, is that she brought in not just Black babies but also white babies. One of the sources of this information came to me from the granddaughter of one of the people my grandmother brought in.

We have a picture that we think was taken after my mother visited Dr. Sherod Chambers. My great-grandmother assisted his wife at birth. We know that because Dr. Chambers kept a journal, and there is a page dedicated to the birthing of Sherod Chambers Jr., who became the surveyor for Hampton.

> *He wrote in his journal, "I went to get Rosa" at such*
> *and such a time. So that was my great-grandmother. The*
> *next installment in the journal was the time of birth.*

Brown also described how family members and Black women who were elders in his church told him about his grandmother's holistic care. Like midwives on the Continent, his great-great-grandmother was much more than a birth attendant.

> BROWN: *They began to care for the expectant mother early on in their pregnancy. Elders at my church and members of my family told me about how my great-grandmother carried what she called a fussing bag. In that context, fussing meant to make a big to-do over you.*
> *They told me how my great-grandmother would come in and massage the stomach and do whatever was needed to make you comfortable. And it was this act of fussing that made the care they received different from going to the doctor. That kind of care kept midwives in play for quite a while.*
> *Midwives were on par with the doctors in birthing work for years until the white doctors specializing in obstetrics and pediatrics moved the midwives on out of it.*

As my conversation with Brown ended, I laughed as I told him that maybe we could form the first international organization of midwife descendants. I explained that I had recently learned from my cousin Sameera Thurmond, a genealogist, that I had a midwife on my family tree. Born in Edgefield, South Carolina, in 1866, Leanna Thurmond Prescott is a distant cousin who attended Shady Grove Baptist Church, the same church my grandparents and great-grandparents attended.

And not far from my community, I met yet another midwife descendant, Maria Valentine. Valentine explained how her grandmother—known to the family as Mama Alice and to the community as Miss Alice—after receiving her lay-midwife permit, cared not only for mothers during childbirth but also for the sick and dying. Living in Portsmouth, Miss Alice also served as the nurse at her church. On Saturday nights, Miss Alice strengthened family bonds among the women in the family, who she invited "to gather on Saturdays to make music by beating on homemade instruments such as cellophane covered hair combs and pots and pans for drums. This was their way to keep the music their forefathers in Africa had passed on to them," Valentine explained. When her grandmother died, Valentine said, her daughter was surprised to see so many people lined up on both sides of the street paying respect to her great-grandmother.

✳

Just as I was finishing this book, I watched Queen Latifah, the groundbreaking rapper and renowned actor, as she learned about her fifth great-grandmother, Juggy Owens, on Henry Louis Gates's television show, *Finding Your Roots*. A free Negro and midwife, Juggy (ca. 1766–1834), lived in Browntown, a community established prior to the Civil War by "Free Negroes" in Princess Ann County, now Virginia Beach, less than 40 miles from where I live. I had an opportunity to visit the Nimmo United Methodist Church near Browntown, where I found out that one of Juggy's descendants might have been an unsung midwife serving in the Union Army Hospital set up in this church.

Kolleda Alexandra, archivist at Fort Monroe, believes that untold midwife stories are buried in Civil War–era muster rolls where Black women, who could have been hired as a laundress, a cook, or a nurse, also served as midwives at Army hospitals during the Civil War era.

A report by surgeon George E. Cooper of the US Army provides a professional view of the efficacy of the Black midwives' work. Although Dr. Cooper refers to midwives as "Negresses," a derogatory term, his report debunks the widely touted medical assessments popularized in the early 20th century. It shows that the Black women who served as midwives in the Old Point Comfort and "adjacent counties" performed their services with extraordinary skill and with rare assistance from an "educated" physician.

✳

Midwives on the Continent describe how birth is the rebirthing of an ancestor whose spirit is eventually recognized and named by a traditional healer, midwife, or elder based on the time the infant was born, the season of the year, or a sound made by the newborn—like a sneeze—that reminds them of a family member who has passed. Now, at Fort Monroe when I take early morning walks, my rituals of remembrance include being mindful of midwife traditions returning like an ancestor being reborn.

Unearthing Black Midwife Stories

I am ending this book with a call to continue the work of collecting the stories of traditional midwives. Although many of
the midwives I interviewed in this book are no longer alive, the
good news is that the women Black midwives cared for, midwife
descendants, and some of the last Black midwives to be licensed
as lay midwives in the 1970s are still alive. I am urging that we
record the stories of these women, as well as others, as soon as
possible.

I know of only one community marker where I live in
Hampton Roads that celebrates the life and work of a midwife.
At the beginning of the 19th century, census records indicate
that there were 600 Black women who identified themselves
as midwives in Elizabeth City County, which included the
city that is now known as Hampton. When will the contributions of Black midwives be recognized on community markers
and become known to tourists on Black history tours? Black
midwives deserve their own tangible markers on the Virginia
landscape.

Statistics from the mid-20th century show us that many
Black elders still living today were brought into the world by
midwives. As recently as 1941, eight years before I was born,

most Black babies in Virginia were born at home. According to Virginia statistics, only 13.7 percent of non-white babies, the term used to refer to Black mothers as well as others, were born in a hospital (I love capitalizing *Black* after decades of statisticians labeling Blacks by describing who we are not versus who we are!). That meant that the overwhelming majority of Black women gave birth at home with midwives. That same year, 45.8 percent of white babies were born in the hospital, and less than 10 percent received care from a midwife.

That same year in Alabama, Mississippi, South Carolina, Georgia, and Florida, two-thirds of Blacks were born at home and attended by midwives. When I interviewed midwives in Alabama in 1981, several of them spoke about how Black midwifery practices were "winding up." That year, when I accompanied Bey Moten, a midwife, to her Alabama church, where she sold her homegrown watermelons after service in the parking lot, I first heard the song "Time Is Winding Up." That song would be the perfect soundtrack for a documentary about the elimination of traditional Black midwife practices across the South in the 1970s. But the good news is that there are still mothers who can describe the care they received from Black midwives in their communities.

✳

Because we can trace Black midwife practices back to the first enslaved Africans to arrive in the colonial period, collecting the stories of Black midwives must also include archival research. For example, Phebe Jackson, a 19th-century Black midwife, healer, and lucrative businesswoman of Petersburg, Virginia, kept records of her caregiving in an account book.

At the University of Virginia Small Library Archives, I held Jackson's only known midwife account book, dated from 1837 to 1846. My hand trembled while slowly turning the fragile, yellowing pages. I also read several plantation account books kept by white men where midwives were referred to by their first name or simply as "midwife." When I saw how Phebe Jackson filled the blank pages in her account book with her first and last names, I smiled, believing that this formerly enslaved woman wanted anyone reading her account book to know that this midwife and healer, who also practiced cupping and bloodletting, a common practice among medical doctors at the time, was independent and free.

Jane Minor, a Black woman who purchased and emancipated Jackson, is believed to have arranged for her apprenticeship to begin her medical and midwifery practices as a businesswoman in Petersburg. Jackson's record book did see the light of day while on display at an exhibition at the Virginia Museum of History and Culture—"Determined: The 400-Year Struggle for Black Equality."

We need to collect and preserve the stories of Black midwives through archival research and oral history, ideally as a midwife story collection project. For example, students at Virginia State University, a Historically Black University in Petersburg, might be interested in learning more about Jackson and collecting other stories of midwives who lived in Petersburg, a community that is less than a 30-minute drive from downtown Richmond. The work of collecting midwife stories begins with documenting practices in the era of enslavement and can include the stories of midwives practicing now. Some Historically Black Colleges and Universities in Virginia have preserved images of Black midwives who participated in health department training programs that Virginia State and Hampton Institute hosted in the 1930s and '40s. Can we create the sites of remembrance where midwives studied, lived, and worked? What can we do to make the stories of Black midwives more visible? In a February 1, 2022, *Time* magazine article, "Black History Lives in Memories and Minds: COVID-19 Has Endangered Those Traditions," Janell Ross illuminates the urgent need to gather the stories of birth workers and midwives. Ross warns: "Recipes passed down through the generations but never written down will never be cooked again."

✳

The idea of launching a project to encourage continuing the collecting and telling of historic Black midwife stories came out of telephone conversation with Dr. Rochanda Mitchell, the last person I interviewed for this book. Just weeks after returning from interviewing midwives on the Continent, I heard Dr. Mitchell on an early Sunday-morning public radio talk show, where she was joined by midwives and doulas who talked about how they were engaged in campaigns to increase birthing justice for Black women.

More than a year later, I caught up with Dr. Mitchell, who had just completed a fellowship in maternal-fetal medicine at the University of Virginia in Charlottesville. The afternoon that we chatted by phone, Dr. Mitchell mentioned that it was her 39th birthday and that it was a good time to talk because her infant was taking an afternoon nap. I smiled about the serendipity but said, "No worries. I'm a grandmother." I insisted that we ended our conversation the moment the baby woke up!

Mitchell joined the medical faculty at Howard University's Department of Obstetrics and Gynecology because of her interest in serving Black women, who are at the highest risk of suffering from health disparities and facing inequities when seeking health care. During her earlier residency at Howard University, Dr. Mitchell's research focused on the impact of food deserts, gestational diabetes, and obesity, conditions that many Black women experience during pregnancy and at birth.

Similar to midwives I interviewed on the Continent and in Alabama, Dr. Mitchell did not need to take a course in cultural competency to learn how to enhance communication and create relationships of mutual trust with the Black patients seeking care at Howard or at UVA in Charlottesville. Like midwives, Dr. Mitchell will be serving mothers who may share similar life experiences. "I come from the back roads of Tennessee. When I see a Black patient, I see my family," Mitchell said. "I know where she is coming from in a literal sense. I am going to take that into consideration as her physician." She continued, "It's hard to provide appropriate care if you can't relate. For some patients, you have to establish rapport before you can go in and tell them what you think is best in caring for their bodies as well as their own lives. I know that I have that gift."

Midwives in Alabama, Africa, and Virginia also said that they had the gift. Dr. Mitchell, however, said she knew little about the practices and traditions of Black midwives and wanted to learn more.

"Where can I learn more about the midwife stories that you and others have collected?" Dr. Mitchell asked.

And that question sparked the idea of encouraging others to collect Black midwife stories now.

Talking to Dr. Mitchell also reminded me that the idea of collecting stories about Black midwives is not just a history project—these stories need to be collected because they include examples of practices that could benefit women now. In spite of depicting Black midwives as "ignorant and backwards," some newspapers published stories that countered negative stereotypes and images. For example, Dr. J. N. Baker, a state health officer in Alabama, reported in 1941 that Black midwives attended two-thirds of Black births, yet Alabama was among the seven states in the nation where "the infant mortality rate for Negroes was slightly less than the national average."

When Dr. Mitchell asked where she could find midwife stories to read, I answered by suggesting that she might start with returning to her home community in the backwoods of Tennessee, where she can sit down at the kitchen table or meet up with elders on a front porch for a conversation about midwives who might have served her community as recently as the 1960s. Dr. Mitchell might find, in having these conversations, that there are practices that could be integrated into caring for Black mothers today in Washington, DC.

Thanks to efforts of communities and organizations over the decades and the momentum of the Black Lives Matter movement, outdoor spaces that once celebrated white supremacy and white privilege are newly liberated community spaces that could become places for staging the stories of Black midwives in communities where they lived and worked. Maybe we could use these spaces to construct a birthing center designed by midwives that has historic images of Black midwives. We could build a café promoting teas and other plant-based medicines recommended by midwives and by the Mampong Centre for Plant Medicine Research in Mampong-Akwapim, Ghana. It would be a space for gardens for relaxation, chanting invocations, praying, meditating, and practicing yoga and other stress-reduction practices. My niece Zetta did yoga headstands the day before having a positive birth experience guided by a midwife in the midst of the COVID pandemic.

Now that I know that there is an ancestor who assisted birthing mothers in Edgefield, South Carolina, I will be calling the genealogist in my family to ask for help in digging up her story. While writing this book, I learned that the heartfelt welcoming I received from midwives as a stranger was just a taste of what these midwives gave to the birthing mothers they knew. Finding a midwife in my own family provided an example of how prevalent midwives continued to be in the Black community. And now, a growing number of midwives and doulas are finding strength and guidance in the traditional practices of midwives on the Continent and in the diaspora similar to the ones included in this book. Writing this book and sharing the experiences of midwives on the Continent and in the diaspora has inspired a new mission in me: to encourage others to find and tell the stories of the midwives of their families, ancestors, and communities. Recognizing the centuries of contributions of Black midwives is long overdue.

Let's build on these stories and make new ones as we move forward in giving strength to the birthing justice movement.

ACKNOWLEDGMENTS

I wish I could compose a jazz suite, choreograph a dance, or create a huge collage to express my gratitude to the countless individuals who contributed to the writing of this book.

I always will be thankful for Khadijah Ishaq, Charles Robertson, and Leola Robertson, who were the first to welcome me to Selma, Alabama, decades ago.

In Nairobi, Kenya, where my work interviewing midwives in Africa began, Kathryn and Penangnini Toure invited me to stay as their guest in a fully furnished apartment filled with sunrising warmth. Also, thank you, Esther Anono, for embracing the Kenya project, and thanks to William C. Notie for assistance in Baringo County.

Frances Ganges, midwife and past International Confederation chief executive, spent countless hours helping me map out a plan for my work on the Continent. I met Frances in the 1970s when she was a student in the cultural competency class that I taught in the nurse midwife program at the University of Medicine and Dentistry of New Jersey. Frances introduced me to Lynn Sibley, a nurse midwife who spent years working within the Ethiopian health care system, and to Dr. Abebe Agebremariam and his wife, Meseret, a nurse midwife. While I was in Addis, Carolyn Curtis, a nurse midwife with years of public health experience, invited me to be a guest in her home.

I also am grateful that in Wolaita Sodo, Ethiopia, Netsanet Abera, at the School of Public Health, Hawassa University, spent countless hours arranging for interviews and interpretation services.

While I was in Ghana, Gertrude Nancy Annan-Aidoo and her family welcomed me into their household in ways that made me feel like I was returning home.

In Northern Ghana, not only did Jennifer Dokbila Mengba and Tikka Winner provide assistance, in our one day of fieldwork in the village of Kpana, we became friends. We also began brainstorming about plans for affiliating with the University of Ghana to make a midwife documentary!

I am grateful that in Ghana, Kenya, and Ethiopia, countless midwives placed babies in my arms for me to hold. It was one of the many ways that I felt I was receiving a blessing.

And I am thankful for the children whose names I will never know who secretly danced with me before dawn in Afar Ethiopia as an Islamic priest's calls to prayer became an invitation to dance.

Teresa Jackson Price and Clarine Baltrip Roberts, both nonagenarians, introduced me to friends who led to my interviewing midwife descendants in Virginia during the COVID pandemic. Thanks to Chardé Reid, Willa Cofield, Julia Dorsey Loomis, and Lisa Hart for reading early drafts. Hugs to Laurie A. Nziah Jefferson, Louis Massiah, April Taylor, Aishah Shahidah Simmons, and others who cheered me along the way. Kwabena Ampofo-Anti—thanks for guiding my work in Ghana. Also thanks to Stoel Markes, raised by his grandmother, Viola Murray, a midwife in Jamaica, who helped to keep me on track.

A special hug for Remica Bigham-Risher, poet and essayist, who mapped out the nine-month plan for our monthly Zoom meetings when COVID put an end to our in-person conversations. Remica's brilliance and energy kept the project alive up to the final birthing of this book.

Regina Rush, Reference Librarian of the Small Special Collections Library at the University of Virginia, became my guiding light in helping me to uncover the stories of eighteenth- and nineteenth-century midwives in Virginia. Sarah E. Thomas provided valuable editing assistance and advice in helping me prepare the manuscript for publication. And I am grateful to Kristen Elias Rowley, editor at The Ohio State University Press, who championed this project even before I interviewed midwives in Africa and Virginia.

The influence of Toni Cade Bambara, writer/cultural worker and friend, is singular because Toni is the first person I discussed this project with. My beloved friend died in 1996, but her spirit lives on in this work. Toni encouraged me to see this project as much more than a book of collated midwife stories. A visionary, Toni suggested that when sitting down with midwives to record their stories, I should talk about organizing a Black midwives union!

Decades ago, Mary Smith Howard, my maternal grandmother, told me stories about the midwives in Uttingertown, a Black community established by previously enslaved members of my family. About midwives who assisted women in the decades following the Civil War, "Mama" said those midwives were "right smart."

It is my family members who deserve a special thank you for seeing me through to the finish line. My daughter, Ghana Smith, at the age of four came in tow to my first Alabama midwife interview. Over the decades that followed, I relentlessly tapped into my daughter's unwavering assistance, depth of spirit, imagination, and brilliance in getting the work done. Keshawn Everett, my grandson, now 23, has always known me as the grandmother immersed in collecting and writing stories about midwives. Beginning in his preschool years, Keshawn helped me keep my balance as he was persistent in inviting me to sit down, go out for meals, and play. My immediate family's thoughtfulness and love carried this book into the light of day.

BIBLIOGRAPHY

Adinew, Yohannes Mehretie, Netsanet Abera Assefa, and Yimenu Mehretie Adinew. "Why Do Some Ethiopian Women Give Birth at Home after Receiving Antenatal Care? Phenomenological Study." *BioMed Research International* 2018 (July 2018). https://doi.org/10.1155/2018/3249786.

Ahmed, Mohammed, Meaza Demissie, Alemayehu Worku, Araya Abrha, and Yamane Barhane. "Socio-cultural Factors Favoring Home Delivery in Afar Pastoral Community, Northeast Ethiopia: A Qualitative Study." *Reproductive Health* 16, no. 171 (November 2019). https://doi.org/10.1186/s12978-019-0833-3.

Akyea, E. Ofori. *Ewe.* New York: Rosen Publishing Group, 1998.

Awolalu, J. Omosade. *Yoruba Beliefs & Sacrificial Rites.* Brooklyn, NY: Athelia Henrietta Press, 1996.

Aziato, Lydia, and Chephas N. Omenyo. "Initiation of Traditional Birth Attendants and Their Traditional and Spiritual Practices During Pregnancy and Childbirth in Ghana." *BMC Pregnancy and Childbirth* 18, no. 64 (March 2018). https://doi.org/10.1186/s12884-018-1691-7.

Badejoko, O. O., H. M. Ibrahim, I. O. Awowole, S. B. Bola-Oyebamiji, A. O. Ijarotimi, and O. M. Loto. "Upright or Dorsal? Childbirth Positions among Antenatal Clinic Attendees in Southwestern Nigeria." *Tropical Journal of Obstetrics Gynecology* 33, no. 2 (January 2016): 172–78. https://doi.org/10.4103/0189-5117.192219.

Bailey, Zizi D., Nancy Krieger, Madina Agénor, Jasmine Graves, Natalia Linos, and Mary T. Bassett. "Structural Racism and Health Inequities in the USA: Evidence and Interventions." *The Lancet* 389, no. 10077 (April 2017): 1453–63. https://doi.org/10.1016/S0140-6736(17)30569-X.

Bassett, Mary T., and Sandro G. Galea. "Reparations as a Public Health Priority: A Strategy for Ending Black-White Health Disparities." *The New England Journal of Medicine* 383, no. 22 (October 2020): 2101–3.

Burnett, Claude A., III, J. A. Jones, J. Rooks, C. H. Chen, C. W. Tyler, and C. A. Miller. "Home Delivery and Neonatal Mortality in North Carolina." *JAMA* 224, no. 24 (December 1980): 2741–45.

Cavanaugh, Dan. "UVA and the History of Race: Confronting Labor Discrimination." *UVA Today,* March 18, 2021. https://news.virginia.edu/content/uva-and-history-race-confronting-labor-discrimination.

Chamberlain, Catherine, Doseena Fergie, Amanda Sinclair, and Christine Asmar. "Traditional Midwifery or 'Wise Women' Models of Leadership: Learning from Indigenous Cultures: '. . . *Lead so the mother is helped, yet still free and in charge . . .*' Lao Tzu, 5th Century BC." *Leadership* 12, no. 3 (July 2016): 346–63. https://doi.org/10.1177%2F1742715015608426.

Chinwe, Nwoye. "An Ethnographic Study of Igbo Naming Ceremony (IBA NWA AFA)." *International Journal of Sociology and Anthropology* 6, no. 10 (October 2014): 276–95. https://doi.org/10.5897/IJSA2014.0529.

De Jonge, Ank, Marlies E. B. Rijnders, Mariet Th. van Diem, Peer L. H. Scheepers, and Antoine L. M. Lagro-Janssen. "Are There Inequalities in Choice of Birthing Position? Sociodemographic and Labour Factors Associated with the Supine Position during the Second Stage of Labour." *Midwifery* 25, no. 4 (August 2009): 439–48. https://doi.org/10.1016/j.midw.2007.07.013.

Duhl, Leonard J., and Nancy Jo Steetle. "Newark: Community or Chaos: A Case Study of the Medical School Controversy." *The Journal of Applied Behavioral Science* 5, no. 4 (December 1969): 537–72. https://doi.org/10.1177/002188636900500406.

Fairhead, James R. "Termites, Mud Daubers and Their Earths: A Multispecies Approach to Fertility and Power in West Africa." *Conservation & Society* 14, no. 4 (2016): 359–67. https://www.jstor.org/stable/26393258?seq=1.

Fett, Sharla M. *Working Cures: Healing Health, and Power on Southern Slave Plantations.* Chapel Hill: University of North Carolina Press, 2002.

Franklin, Rosy C., Ryan A. Behmer Hansen, Jean M. Pierce, Diomedes J. Tsitouras, and Catherine A. Mazzola. "Broken Promises to the People of Newark: A Historical Review of the Newark Uprising, the Newark Agreements, and Rutgers New Jersey Medical School's Commitments to Newark." *International Journal of Environmental Research and Public Health* 18, no. 4 (February 2021): Article 2117. https://doi.org/10.3390/ijerph18042117.

Fraser, Gertrude Jacinta. *African American Midwifery in the South: Dialogues of Birth, Race,* and *Memory.* Cambridge, MA: Harvard University Press, 1998.

Galbraith, Robert. *Reclaiming Midwives: Stills from "All My Babies."* San Francisco: 81 Press, 2005.

Greenwood, Brad N., Rachel R. Hardeman, Laura Huang, and Aaron Sojourner. "Physician–Patient Racial Concordance and Disparities in Birthing Mortality for Newborns." *Proceedings of the National Academy of Sciences of the United States of America* 117, no. 35 (August 2020): 21194–200. https://doi.org/10.1073/pnas.1913405117.

Greenfield, Eloise. *The Women Who Caught the Babies: A Story of African American Midwives.* Carrboro, NC: Alazar Press, 2019.

Grindal, Bruce T. "An Ethnographic Classification of the Sisala of Northern Ghana." *Ethnography* 11, no. 4 (October 1972): 409–24. https://doi.org/10.2307/3773072.

Grundy, Saida. "The False Promise of Anti-racism Books." *The Atlantic,* July 21, 2020. https://www.theatlantic.com/culture/archive/2020/07/your-anti-racism-books-are-means-not-end/614281/.

Hoffman, Kelly M., Sophie Trawalter, Jordan R. Axt, and M. Norman Oliver. "Racial Bias in Pain Assessment and Treatment: Recommendations and False Beliefs about Biological Differences between Blacks and Whites." *Proceedings of the National Association of Science of the United States of America* 113, no. 16 (April 2016): 4296–301. https://doi.org/10.1073/pnas.1516047113.

Holland, Endesha Ida Mae. *From the Mississippi Delta.* New York: Simon and Schuster, 1997.

Holmes, Linda Janet. "Alabama Granny Midwives." *Journal of the Medical School of New Jersey* 81 (1984): 389–91.

Holmes, Linda Janet. *Into the Light of Day: Reflections on the History of Midwives of Color within the American College of Nurse-Midwives.* Silver Spring, MD: American College of Nurse-Midwives, 2012.

———. "Thank You Jesus to Myself: The Life of a Traditional Black Midwife." In *The Black Women's Health Book: Speaking for Ourselves,* edited by Evelyn C. White, 98–106. Seattle, WA: Seal Press, 1990.

Holmes, Linda Janet, and Louvenia Taylor Benjamin. "Southern Lay Midwife: An Interview." *Sage: A Scholarly Journal on Black Women* 2, no. 2 (Fall 1985): 51–54.

Hunter, John M. "Macroterme Geophagy and Pregnancy Clays in Southern Africa." *Journal of Cultural Geography* 14, no. 1 (1993): 69–92. https://doi.org/10.1080/08873639309478381.

Kahn, Robbie. *Bearing Meaning: The Language of Birth.* Urbana and Chicago: University of Illinois Press, 1995.

Kirui, E., G. Nguka, J. Wango, G. O. Abong, and G. Muchemi. "Factors That Negatively Influence Consumption of Traditionally Fermented Milk (Mursik) among Preschool Children (1–5 years old) in Kapseret Location-Uasin Gishu County, Kenya." *African Journal of Food, Agriculture, Nutri-*

tion, and Development 17, no. 3 (July 2017): 12295–310. https://ajfand.net/Volume17/No3/Kirui16005.pdf.

Kitila, Sena Belina, Wondwosen Molla, Tilahun Wedaynewu, Tadele Yadessa, and Melikamu Gellan. "Folk Practice during Childbirth and Reasons for the Practice in Ethiopia: A Systematic Review." *Gynecology & Obstetrics* 8, no. 3 (March 2018). https://doi.org/10.4172/2161-0932.1000465. Available at https://www.longdom.org/open-access/folkpracticeduring-childbirth-and-reasons-for-the-practice-in-ethiopia-asystematic-review-2161-0932-1000465.pdf.

Kitzinger, Sheila. *Rediscovering Birth.* New York: Pocket Books, 2001.

Kwame, Abukari. "An Ethnographic Sketch of Social Interaction in Dagbon Society: The Case of Greeting, Sharing Drinks and Kola Nut." *Journal of Multidisciplinary Resources at Trent* 2, no. 1 (December 2019): 1–20.

Loan, Onnie Lee, as told to Katherine Clark. *Motherwit: An Alabama Midwife's Story.* New York: E. P. Dutton, 1989.

Mawoza, Tariro, Charles Nhachi, and Thulani Magwali. "Prevalence of Traditional Medicine Use during Pregnancy, at Labour and for Postpartum Care in a Rural Area in Zimbabwe." *Clinics in Mother and Child Health* 16, no. 2 (April 2019): Article 321. https://doi.org/10.24105/2090-7214.16.321.

McKay, Nellie. "An Interview with Toni Morrison." *Contemporary Literature* 24, no. 4 (Winter 1983): 413–29.

Mbiti, John S. *African Religions and Philosophy.* New York: Anchor Books, Doubleday, 1969.

Muigai, Wangui. "'Something Wasn't Clean': Black Midwifery, Birth, and Postwar Medical Education in *All My Babies*." *Bulletin of the History of Medicine* 93, no. 1 (2019): 82–113. https://doi.org/10.1353/bhm.2019.0003.

Musie, Maurine R., Mmapheko D. Peu, and Warshika Bahana-Pema. "Factors Hindering Midwives' Utilisation of Alternative Birth Positions during Labour in a Selected Public Hospital." *African Journal of Primary Health Care & Family Medicine* 11, no. 1 (September 2019): e1–e8. https://doi.org/10.4102/phcfm.v11i1.2071.

Muthiani, Joseph. *Akamba from Within: Egalitarianism in Social Relations.* New York: Exposition Press, 1973.

Nelson, Louis P., and Claudrena N. Harold, eds. *Charlottesville 2017: The Legacy of Race and Inequity.* Charlottesville: University of Virginia Press, 2018.

"NHIF's 'Linda Mama' Program Reduces Infant Mortality Rates in Baringo." *NTV News, Nation,* April 22, 2018. https://nation.africa/kenya/videos/news/nhif-s-linda-mama-program-reduces-infant-mortality-rates-in-baringo-1260812 (accessed June 9, 2022).

Nijiru, Haron, Uriel Elchalal, and Ora Paltiel. "Geophagy during Pregnancy in Africa: A Literature Review." *Obstetrical and Gynecological Survey* 66, no. 7 (July 2011): 452–57. https://doi.org/10.1097/OGX.0b013e318232a034.

Niles, P. Mimi, and Michelle Drew. "Constructing the Modern American Midwife: White Supremacy and White Feminism Collide." *Nursing Clio*, October 22, 2020. https://nursingclio.org/2020/10/22/constructing-the-modern-american-midwife-white-supremacy-and-white-feminism-collide/.

Oketch, Angela. "Linda Mama Has Received Over Sh13bn, Says PS." *Nation*, July 24, 2021. https://nation.africa/kenya/news/linda-mama-has-received-over-sh13bn-says-ps-3484472.

Olupona, Jacob K., ed. *African Traditional Religions in Contemporary Society*. St. Paul, MN: Paragon House, 1991.

Oparah, Julia Chinyere, and Alicia D. Bonaparte, eds. *Birthing Justice: Black Women, Pregnancy, and Childbirth*. New York: Routledge, 2016.

Owens, Deirdre Cooper. *Medical Bondage: Race, Gender, and the Origins of American Gynecology*. Athens: University of Georgia Press, 2017.

Peprah, Prince, Emmanuel Mawuli Abalo, Julius Nyonyo, Reforce Okwei, Williams Agyemang-Duah, and Godfred Amankwaa. "Pregnant Women's Perception and Attitudes Toward Modern and Traditional Midwives and the Perceptional Impact on Health Seeking Behaviour and Status in Rural Ghana." *International Journal of African Nursing Sciences* 8 (March 2018): 66–74. https://doi.org/10.1016/j.ijans.2018.03.003.

Roberson, Joshua. "The Early History of 'New Kingdom' Netherworld Iconography: A Late Middle Kingdom Apotropaic Wand Reconsidered." In *Archaism and Innovation: Studies in the Culture of Middle Kingdom Egypt*, edited by David P. Silverman, William Kelly Simpson, and Josef W. Wegner, 427–96. New Haven, CT: Department of Near Eastern Languages and Civilizations, Yale University, 2009.

Robinson, Karina, and Caitlin Hogan. "Childbirth in Ancient Egypt: Nature's Unique Work of Art." *Probe Magazine*, June 27, 2018. https://www.ssbprobe.com/articles/childbirth-in-egypt.

Smith, Margaret Charles, and Linda Janet Holmes. *Listen to Me Good: The Life Story of an Alabama Midwife*. Columbus: The Ohio State University Press, 1996.

Sonkin, Robert, and Annie Shamburger. *Annie Shamburger, Project Nurse, Talking about Health*. Recorded in Gee's Bend, Alabama, 1941. American Folklife Center, Library of Congress. https://www.loc.gov/item/afc9999005.14440/.

Taylor-Guthrie, Danille Kathleen, ed. *Conversations with Toni Morrison*. Jackson: University Press of Mississippi, 1994.

Turner, Sasha. *Contested Bodies: Pregnancy, Childrearing, and Slavery in Jamaica*. Philadelphia: University of Pennsylvania Press, 2017.

University of Pennsylvania. "Archaeologists Uncover 3700-Year-Old 'Magical' Birth Brick in Egypt." *EurekAlert!* July 25, 2002. https://www.eurekalert.org/news-releases/820261.

Vedam, Saraswathi, Kathrin Stoll, Marian MacDorman, Eugene Declercq, Renee Cramer, Melissa Cheyney, Timothy Fisher, Emma Butt, Y. Tony Yang, and Holly Powell Kennedy. "Mapping Integration of Midwives across the United States: Impact on Access, Equity and Outcomes." *PLOS One* 13, no. 2 (February 2018). https://doi.org/10.1371/journal.pone.0192523.

Wegner, Josef. "The Archaeology of South Abydos: Egypt's Late Middle Kingdom in Microcosm." *Expedition Magazine* 48, no. 2 (2006). https://www.penn.museum/sites/expedition/the-archaeology-of-south-abydos/.

————. "A Decorated Birth-Brick from South Abydos: New Evidence on Childbirth and Birth Magic in the Middle Kingdom," in *Archaism and Innovation: Studies in the Culture of Middle Kingdom Egypt*, edited by David P. Silverman, William Kelly Simpson, and Josef W. Wegner, 447-96. New Haven, CT: Department of Near Eastern Languages and Civilizations, Yale University, 2009.

————. "The Magical Birth Brick." *Expedition Magazine* 48, no. 2 (2006). https://www.penn.museum/sites/expedition/the-magical-birth-brick/.

Wells-Oghoghomeh, Alexis. *The Souls of Womenfolk: The Religious Cultures of Enslaved Women in the Lower South.* Chapel Hill: University of North Carolina Press, 2021.

WHO Reproductive Health Library. "WHO Recommendation on Respectful Maternity Care during Labour and Childbirth." *World Health Organization,* February 15, 2018. https://srhr.org/rhl/article/who-recommendation-on-respectful-maternity-care-during-labour-and-childbirth.

Wilkie, Laurie A. *The Archaeology of Mothering: An African-American Midwife's Tale.* New York: Routledge, 2003.

Young, Sera L. *Craving Earth: Understanding Pica: The Urge to Eat Clay, Starch, Ice & Chalk.* New York: Columbia University Press, 2011.

INDEX

Aaron, Mary, 100–102, 122

adowa (antelope) dance, 76–77

Adzorhlor, Mama, III, 119–20

Afar, Ethiopia: about, 39–40, 44–45; coffee ceremony, 48; Fatuma Hamadu, 46–47; Hawa Galali Elissa, 40–41; Mariam Awwol Mohammed, 45–48; Momina Abdalla Mussa, 42–44; Udama Ali Mohammed, 40–42

Africatown, Mobile, AL, 125–26, 129, 133–37, 145

afterbirth. *See* placenta burial

Aidoo, Gertrude Annan, 65–66, 76–77

Akoto, Baffour Osei, xvii–xviii

Akufo-Addo, Nana, 1

Akyea, E. Ofori, 77

Alabama: Alabama prohibition against plant medicines, 99–100; civil rights movement in, 95, 107–9; elimination of lay midwives in, 79–80; Bey Moten, 170. *See also* Mobile, AL; Montgomery, AL; Selma, AL

Alabama Health Department, 99–101, 108

Alexandra, Kolleda, 167

Allen, Pollee, 133

American College of Nurse-Midwives Truth and Reconciliation Task Force, 161

Ampofo, Oku, 74

ancestors, 19–20, 56–57, 62–63

ancestral spirits returning in birth, 59–60

Angelou, Maya, 51

apprenticeship: in Lowndes County, AL, 100; in Montgomery, AL, 83, 86; in Wolaita Sodo, Ethiopia, 32

Ashanti Kingdom, 51, 65–66

ashes, sweeping or carrying out, 114, 118, 121

Ayelech Hafamo, 34–37

Baformene, Hoya, 66, 70–73, 75–76

Baker, J. N., 173

Baringo County, Kenya: about, 13–14; Kamia, 21–25; Khadijah, 14–15, 25–26; Makena, 19–21; Rachael, 15–17; Susan, 17–19

Barrett, Roberta, 153

185

ABOUT THE AUTHOR

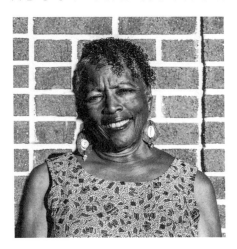

Linda Janet Holmes is an independent scholar, the former director of New Jersey's Office of Minority and Multicultural Health,
and a women's health activist. Her writing—including articles
in medical and feminist journals—has contributed to a resur-
gence of international recognition of the significance of African American midwifery practices. She is the coauthor (with
Margaret Charles Smith) of *Listen to Me Good: The Story of an
Alabama Midwife,* author of *A Joyous Revolt: Toni Cade Bambara, Writer and Activist,* and coeditor (with Cheryl A. Wall) of
Savoring the Salt: The Legacy of Toni Cade Bambara. She lives in
Hampton, Virginia.